Also by Donna Jackson Nakazawa

Does Anybody Else Look Like Me?
The Last Best Cure
The Autoimmune Epidemic
Childhood Disrupted
The Angel and the Assassin
Girls on the Brink
The Adverse Childhood Experiences Guided Journal

Mind Drama

Mind Drama

The Science of Rumination and How to Outwit Your Inner Defeatist

Donna Jackson Nakazawa

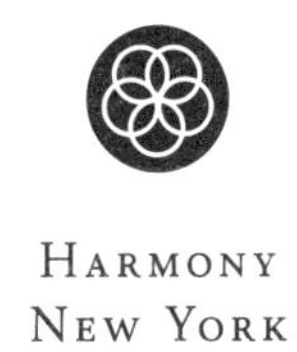

HARMONY
NEW YORK

Harmony Books
An imprint of Random House
A division of Penguin Random House LLC
1745 Broadway, New York, NY 10019
harmonybooks.com | randomhousebooks.com
penguinrandomhouse.com

ISBN 978-0-593-98019-4
Ebook ISBN 978-0-593-98020-0

Printed in the United States of America

1st Printing

First Edition

BOOK TEAM: Production editor: Michelle Daniel • Managing editor: Allison Fox • Production manager: Maggie Hart • Copy editor: Sara Robb • Proofreaders: Andrea Gordon, Barbara Jatkola, Rachel Kirsch

Book design by Kevin Quach

The authorized representative in the EU for product safety and compliance is Penguin Random House Ireland, Morrison Chambers, 32 Nassau Street, Dublin D02 YH68, Ireland.
https://eu-contact.penguin.ie

For Zen, Christian, and Claire

PREFACE

I WAS SITTING in my eye doctor's waiting room when my smartphone rang. The call was from a British scientist I'd known for a while. He'd recently asked to read a manuscript for a book I'd written that was coming out later that year. If he could read it in advance, he'd told me, he could offer feedback. Usually, I wouldn't show anyone my unpublished work, but his offer seemed genuine and well meant, and I'd sent it to him a week or so earlier. What science writer doesn't want feedback from a scientist? It could only make my work better. So I walked out of the waiting room and took his call.

He was, he told me, writing a paper for a research journal. In his paper—he didn't think I'd mind—he'd borrowed key sections from my book that encapsulated my core argument. In a paper under his name.

I struggled to understand. When I'd sent him my manuscript, I'd explicitly said he couldn't use anything he read, especially since my book wouldn't be out for many months. "You can't use material taken from my book! In your paper!"

"Well, now that I've read it, I can't pretend I don't know what I know. You've synthesized recent science to create a significant argument that can help people."

I sputtered on the other end of the phone.

"Besides, don't you want people to have this information sooner? They shouldn't have to wait for your book to come out."

My shock shifted into anger. "You can't publish my work under your name!" My heart hammered in my chest. "When my book comes out, people will think I'm stealing *your* ideas when you're the one taking *my* work."

He talked about the authority his name would lend to my ideas, enabling them to find a wider audience. A creepy sensation made the hairs on the back of my neck prick up—the sensation of being ill-used and gaslit. "I'll have to alert my publisher to your intentions," I told him.

Now he seemed stunned. "You don't need to do *that.* We're friends, aren't we? We can work something out between us, can't we?"

I stabbed my finger at my phone to end the call. My hands were shaking. My mind future-tripped into possible scenarios that might play out. If I fought back, he could do real harm to my career. Fear disintegrated into a thought bomb of self-loathing and regret. *Why did I show him my manuscript? Why did I think I could trust him? I have only myself to blame! What kind of idiot lets something like this happen? I* do, apparently. Self-blame seesawed back to rage. *What kind of person does this to another person? One more old white dude who tries to coerce and take advantage of a woman who holds less status and power than he does!* A familiar dread unfurled in my chest and radiated down through my arms, my legs.

I looked back toward the waiting room. I could not sit through my eye exam in this state.

I told the front desk I was suddenly feeling unwell and needed to reschedule. My fists grew white as I clutched the steering wheel and drove home. Once there, our dogs danced around me, winding their bodies through my legs, snouts nudging me as insistently as did my thoughts about the conversation I'd just had. When I didn't offer both dogs their usual head and belly rubs, they began to chuff with small, worried barks. I called out for my husband, hoping he might hear me from upstairs. My voice did not sound like my own. The dogs barked more.

He came running downstairs and took in my overall state. "Are you okay? My God, your face is red! You're shaking!"

I told him everything.

He advised action. "Email your editor now. You have to let her know what happened."

I logged on to my computer and saw the British researcher had already emailed me. *Whew*, I thought. He must have realized he'd been out of line, way out of line. I opened his email, certain he was writing to apologize. But I was wrong. He was doubling down on his effort to sway me. By letting him use my work, I would get my ideas out there faster and "help more people." It didn't matter whose name it was under. "I *know* you want this, too," he wrote.

I emailed my editor. My body had begun to tremble all over, my chest quaking uncontrollably.

Ten minutes later, her response pinged my inbox. Within the hour, we were on the phone with her legal department, who told me what to do. In the end, the British scientist did not publish my work under his name before my book came out. The whole unhappy incident was resolved within a few hours. Disaster avoided. Nothing more to be said. Just a single day of my life, and it was all behind me now. Over.

But that is not what happened inside my head. The story went on and on, my mind replaying scenes—mental movies only I could see—of what had happened. In each recursive thought loop, I chastised myself, thinking of what I should have said or done differently in the time I'd known the British scientist. Snippets of past conversations, moments in which I'd revealed personal details of my life, thinking I could trust him, came back to me. His words, "I *know* you want this, too," reverberated through my body, reminding me of other times I'd thought I could trust a powerful man and something bad, even terrible, had happened to me. A slew of old beliefs I'd always secretly considered to be true about myself reemerged, blaring their insidious voices. *People don't respect me or my work.*

My voice doesn't matter. No one values what I have to say. My feelings are expendable. I am expendable. This litany infiltrated my mind until it felt like the only real truth about me. I was trapped in my head, and it was a bad neighborhood to be in.

By evening, the emotional fallout from my thought-spiraling had radiated autonomically through every bodily system. My guts emptied. Tingling and numbness in my hands, feet, and face—a neuropathy that lingered from a more serious autoimmune disorder that had at times rendered me critically ill—intensified, as it sometimes did under severe physical or emotional stress. I could not feel my nose when I touched it. My feet were numb in my shoes. This hadn't happened in years. I asked my husband to lie down next to me, shoulder to shoulder, hip to hip, and squeezed his hand, trying to calm myself, hoping my body's rhythm would align with his slower, steadier heartbeat.

I'd like to say that I, who've written more than a half dozen books about the connection between emotion, trauma, and health, was able to slam the brakes on my escalating mind drama. But despite all I knew, despite the meditation and yoga I'd stacked into my day for decades, I could not. In quiet moments—driving, washing dishes, going for a walk—my brain kept bringing me back, my thoughts pinned to those few moments of my life like a butterfly to a board, unable to wrest free.

Eventually, a good friend—a fellow writer who shared my horror and had commiserated with me at length over what had happened—said to me, quite gently, "It happened two weeks ago. You have been ruminating on this too long. It's time to stop. What happened was horribly upsetting and would be for anyone—but I don't think replaying it over and over again is good for you."

Her words struck me. One in particular—*ruminating.* Yes, that's what I was doing. Before the incident with the British researcher, I had already noticed that my lifelong tendency to get sucked into a vortex of obsessive thought had become more prevalent of late. Over the previous year, or two, maybe three—it was hard to pin down—I'd found myself getting caught up in doom-and-gloom thought loops more often than usual. This mental bad-weather pattern had become more habitual, as if my brain had moved into a new climate where it was forever rainy. I felt ten degrees off-kilter: a touch more anxious; a bit more forgetful.

Whenever these disturbing thought ripples played through my mind, scenes and emotions completely unrelated to whatever task I was doing in the moment took center stage. One day, I was ducking my head under the kitchen table to sweep up dog hair and got so wrapped up in replaying the incident with the British researcher that I conked my head on the corner of the table as I stood up. By the next morning, a bruise the color and size of a plum had spread across my temple.

Another day, I was driving my mother home after I'd just run some errands for her when she rattled off yet another to-do list for me to take care of "next time." I was happy to help my mom, I love my mom, but I was also managing deadlines and travel for speaking events, not to mention a few pressing and, of late, more troublesome health issues of my own. When I reminded her that I was working the rest of that week, she said, "But you're my only *daughter*." Suddenly, my mind disappeared into the quicksand of old mental movies—moments in my childhood when I'd had to tend to my mother's waves of despair, grief, and rage, and navigate her confusing outbursts. I was twelve when my father died in a sudden and unimaginable tragedy, and despite my own stunned child's grief, I'd found myself, as the youngest child but the only girl—yes, her only daughter, but not her only child; I had three older brothers—thrust into the role of tending to her moods and needs. I sublimated my own despair, as children do when they feel unseen and afraid. Suddenly ensnared in old scenes and stories from my past as I drove her home that day, I took a wrong turn.

But these were hardly the only times I'd gotten that lost in my thoughts. Just that morning, I'd let our little rescue dog out for a minute, turned around to wash a few dishes before bringing her back in, but became so absorbed in a problem my daughter had confided she was struggling with that I forgot Winnie. Then I went out for a walk, only to look up and find her trotting alongside me on the road, without a leash. This was just not like me. I did not forget such things.

In the end, the incident with the British scientist, because it was so extreme and dramatic, called attention to something inside me that I had been willfully ignoring and needed to examine more closely: my increasing tendency to get lost in my own mind drama to the point that it commandeered too many precious moments of my waking life.

Could I, I wondered, apply my reporting skills to understand my growing tendency to ruminate, and find simple-to-implement, science-based ways to address this unwelcome and draining mental habit? And in so doing, could I help others find relief from their habits of rumination, too?

I knew I wasn't the only one who was suffering. I thought of how recently, the X account for *Sesame Street*'s red furry monster Elmo had posed a simple question to its half million followers: "Elmo is just checking in! How is everybody doing?" Nearly twenty thousand people, most of them adults, responded, many of them telling Elmo they found themselves struggling and lost in despair-laden thoughts. In a quickly released statement, *Sesame Street* execs said they had never anticipated "how deeply this particular question would resonate." No one had expected so much, well, rumination to rear its head in response to a question from a *Sesame Street* puppet!

And so my journey began. For the past twenty-five years, as a science journalist and author of a number of books on the intersection of neuroscience and emotion, I have worked with leading neuroscientists and psychologists to frame workshops and trainings that I deliver all over the country at universities, national organizations, and schools. As I began to wade into the latest annals of science on rumination for this book, this new exploration was no different; I talked to dozens of leading experts in the field, interviewed lots of other people with a penchant for ruminating, and had my own brain scanned to see how much of a ruminator I was.

This mission is one part research, one part me-search. I hope you'll find this book useful, but to be completely honest, I wrote it for myself. I might be guiding you, but I'll also be beside you, learning in lockstep. If you go on this journey with me, I think you'll find that what I've uncovered will help you to turn your life around in ways that will make you calmer, happier, more creative, and more grounded. Ultimately, I think you'll find that you become more *you.* A you that is gentler with yourself.

In this book, you'll learn what I've learned. According to scientists who track mental well-being, we are ruminating more than we ever have before. This is a problem, because the degree to which we ruminate, perhaps more than any other mental act, determines our lifelong well-being. You'll also learn how early life experiences wire up a key part of your brain that gives rise to your ruminations, and why—when triggered by echoes of your difficult life experiences—this brain area goes into lockdown, trapping you in your deepest and most self-deprecating thoughts. In this way, your patterns of rumination—those sticky thought cycles you can't escape—have something profound to tell you; they are signal fires from your past. Once you understand the messages they are sending you, you can effectively reverse engineer them, and by so doing, begin to heal.

No matter who you are or what your story might be, this destructive mental habit of rumination is within your locus of control. With practice, you can learn powerful, science-proven strategies to exit your dark, untamed thoughts. From here, you can learn how to repurpose your brain's ruminative tendencies to access your mind's higher potential for creativity, ingenuity, and insight. Taken together, this will change the tenor and quality of your life.

◆ ◆ ◆ ◆

A few final words on how this book is structured. In most of the chapters, you'll discover what the latest findings from science and psychology reveal about why it's so important to make these powerful shifts in your ruminative behavior, followed by practical techniques road tested by me and by the stalwart individuals who have joined me in this quest. No single technique is a silver bullet, so choose and combine the techniques that resonate with you—those that make you feel more open, more present, free to take delight in yourself and in the world. Let those that you most enjoy seep into your psyche. The more you do, the more readily you'll be able to call upon these strategies when you need them most, and the more change you'll enjoy.

If you are someone who, as I do, loves (maybe even needs) to understand the scientific underpinnings to explain why such actions will be effective, start with part 1. It's all there.

If you need immediate SOS strategies to quell your ruminating thought spirals, jump to parts 2 and 3 for some quick and effective practices to help you do that. You can always come back, when you're ready, to read the earlier chapters for more of the *why* behind the *how-to.* If you are someone dealing with the lingering effects of more pervasive trauma, you will want to move slowly, delving into parts 2 and 3, paying special attention to chapter 12, where we'll touch on severe trauma and a few, very new, science-based ways to get more help. As with any journey that helps you to move toward a deeper emotional engagement with what's been keeping you stuck, be gentle with yourself. Always. And if you ever feel, even for an instant, overwhelmed, reach out for more immediate assistance.

Part 4 will guide you on a journey into the upside of rumination, because believe it or not, there can be an upside. Here, you'll discover how to tap into rumination in a creative, life-enhancing way.

If you aren't quite sure if you have a tendency toward unhealthy rumination, see the appendix, where I offer a ten-minute questionnaire to help you assess your mental habits and discern whether rumination is a problem in your life.

Finally, as you set out to understand and free yourself from your self-defeating ruminations, please don't think of this journey as one more step in a never-ending push for self-improvement. It's not about trying to master, optimize, or conquer any aspect of who you are. By doing this work, I hope you'll come to see that your ruminations hold within them precious pieces of your psyche that are waiting to be seen, brought to light, understood, and, yes, loved. Once you understand and listen to what they have to tell you, you will lighten a heavy, invisible burden that you've been carrying for a very long time. You'll only know how heavy a weight it was once you've set it down.

CONTENTS

I

Where Does Your Mind Drama Come From?

ONE

The Power and Peril of Rumination

I'M SITTING IN a small, dark room, half-office, half-lab, staring at a computer screen showing what looks like a bright red cyclone barreling across scans of my brain. Next to me sits clinical neuroscientist Mark Trullinger, PhD, who uses AI, fMRI-like brain scans, and electrical brain waves to read an individual's brain state as if he's reading their personal biography. Without knowing much about my current life, he's certainly doing a great job of reading mine.

"What is *that*?" I point to the ominous red swirl on the scans of my brain he'd taken at our previous appointment.

"These are little earthquakes of rumination that are erupting all the time in your brain." Trullinger moves his cursor over the scarlet blob. "See here? Some sort of long-standing emotional stress is triggering regular spurts of rumination." He moves the cursor slightly to the right. "And here, I can see that chronic health conditions are triggering more little explosions of rumination." He sits back in his chair and turns to look at me. "The problem is that once this area of the brain becomes hyper-primed, it's very hard for your brain to toggle back out of your ruminating thoughts"—those recursive and distressing thought loops in which so many of us become entangled.

"What area of the brain are we looking at here?"

"The default mode network. This network is the seat of your sense of self. It's also your brain's storyteller, where you spin stories about who you are, how you got here, what's happened to you in your life—and who you can become. Think of it as the birthplace of all the self-referential thoughts that shape how you judge yourself and others." As its name implies, the default mode network *is* a network. It's made up of three brain areas that, together, generate our ruminations: the *posterior cingulate cortex*, which helps us recall our memories; the *dorsal medial prefrontal cortex*, which brings forth our difficult emotions; and the *parietal lobe*, which generates our physical sensations.

Trullinger is a neuroscientist who also practices psychology, which makes him a unicorn in the field. He can examine our brain activity to gain a unique perspective on our hidden emotional life—past, present, and future. Trullinger also serves as the director of NeuroThrive, a clinical practice that assesses individuals' brain function and how to improve it, and sits on the advisory board of the research advocacy group BrainFutures (which, in full disclosure, I also sit on).

The problem, Trullinger continues, is that "when chronic stress levels stay elevated, the brain can shift into prolonged bouts of rumination and get stuck there. And that's not good, because over time this heavy pattern of rumination can lead to anxiety, mood changes, mental fatigue, and years from now, when you're older, memory issues."

Trullinger seems to be reading the tea leaves of my life right now. I stifle the urge to tell him that despite my increased episodes of ruminating, I *am* a normal person, a get-it-done, practical person, someone who has a career I love, and loving relationships with my husband, children, and friends.

Perhaps he sees the consternation fall over my face, because before I can speak, he adds, "You also show some beautiful strengths in your brain." His cursor slides toward another area of my brain, to the posterior cingulate cortex, the part of my default mode network that plays a role in higher-level cognitive functions, including awareness, perception, social cognition, and information integration. "I can see you have an acute ability to make complex associations between abstract ideas in a very deep way—here, your brain is functioning more optimally than the norm. And your perceptual awareness about everything happening around you is unusual. You are probably one of the first people in any room to sense how people are feeling; the first to know when something is off, or if there is danger, if someone needs help. You also show a heightened ability to switch into a positive, productive type of ruminating and mind-wandering—creativity, imagination, ideation."

Because I've become so acutely aware of the ways in which rumination has been draining me, I'm thrilled to hear that there is a positive form of rumination, one that could potentially feed my creativity and yield more moments of insight.

"But once you get stuck in negative recursive thoughts, your brain becomes tired and anxious," he adds. "And it drifts away, shutting out everything but those darker storylines."

Now I'm really worried. "Are you saying I ruminate *more* than other people?"

"Well, that's a tricky question." Trullinger exits out of the images we've been looking at and pulls up several recent research papers. "When we compare people's brains from five years ago, before the pandemic, to today, we can see that people are, in general, more likely to become locked in unhealthy, ruminating thoughts." There are, he says, notable alterations in the default mode network that correlate to our collective hyper-ruminative state. "The pandemic is unlikely to be the only cause, but we do know that something significant has changed."

I consider the overall apocalyptic feel of the world right now. Ideological and political divides that feel uglier, more volatile, and more impassable than ever. A yearslong pandemic that was terrifying only slightly in the rearview mirror. A growing epidemic of loneliness. Too much Zooming, too little in-person connection. The barrage of negative news and discord blaring our way morning, noon, and night. Mass shootings, an unprecedented mental health crisis, the growing disaster of climate change, and several hate-fueled wars. Even traffic fatalities are at their highest levels in decades thanks to unprecedented bouts of road rage. Then there's the dark, addictive rabbit hole of social media, spewing such a fire hose of news and opinions about political events and social turmoil that it requires a constant and exhausting effort to distinguish the real from the fake. The same week I was in Trullinger's office, Oxford University Press had announced that after analyzing language data and holding a public vote in which thirty-seven thousand people participated, their word of the year was *brain rot*, referring to the deleterious effect of consuming too much "low-quality" online content, especially on social media.

It does seem some days like it would be best to pull the covers over one's head or move to an island off Fiji. Could this vitriolic world in which we live be making it harder than ever to stop ruminating about both external events and the problems that plague us in our personal lives?

I share with Trullinger that I already meditate every day, do yoga, take long walks in nature, exercise, see my therapist. "But none of it seems to be quite enough anymore."

"These are excellent things to do. Imagine how much worse it would be if you weren't doing them!" He laughs. "But research shows that as beneficial and important as these are, they may not be enough. People often need additional tools that more directly target rumination."

"Such as?"

"That's one of the hottest topics in neuroscience." During my subsequent meetings with Trullinger, as well as other neuroscientists and psychologists, this was one of the subjects we would explore.

As I leave Trullinger's office that day, I'm even more curious and determined to understand the damage rumination does to our mental health and cognitive clarity, and how we can wrest ourselves free from it. Having heard Trullinger say that rumination can offer something positive, fueling our imagination and our creativity, I also want to know how we can flip the switch and transform our dark ruminative energy into something empowering and purposeful. What can science tell us about the upside of rumination, the creative state of ideation and ingenuity that fills us with joy and an intense, palpable feeling of interior well-being? Clearly the ruminators among us, and apparently there are more of us than ever, need better tactics and strategies to escape our looping thoughts and exchange them for something creative and insightful.

This gives rise to other questions on my mind: How big a problem is rumination, really, for everyone? Is it as widespread as I think, or is it just that I don't want to feel so alone?

When I get home, a search of the recent literature at the National Library of Medicine corroborates what Trullinger already told me. Compared to prior to the pandemic, our brains today are a lot more likely to show not only markers of increased emotional distress but "alterations" in activity in the default mode network—the seat of our ruminating thoughts. And yup, most of us appear to be ruminating more than we did five years ago.

Still, I wonder how this observation resonated with psychologists who treat clients every day. I reach out to psychologist Sally Winston, PsyD, who studies rumination and is the codirector of the Anxiety and Stress Disorders Institute of Maryland. I tell her I'm wondering if my hunch as to why we're all more mired in rumination rings true for her, given her clinical expertise. "It's clear that information and misinformation overload, as well as the deliberate evocation of emotion-laden and fear-provoking content, play a role in why people are ruminating more than they used to," she says. Everything we could possibly stew or worry over is so much more in our face "than was true when we were not being bombarded." Not only are we presented with so much more to worry about, but because we are all so glued to our screens, we're often removed from the human connections and healthier pastimes that ordinarily tether us to reality and help keep us safely out of our heads.

Many Americans are clearly struggling to find emotional and mental relief. Already in 2010, a famous Harvard study found that we spent nearly half our waking hours spinning "neutral" or "unhappy" stories, rather than feeling engaged in the activities we were currently doing. And most of this rumination time—amounting to 26 percent of our waking life—was spent on "unhappy" thoughts. (If we're awake sixteen hours a day, that's four hours a day spent in distressing thoughts.) No one has done a follow-up study to see whether we are spending more than 26 percent of our time in unhappy thought loops today, but other measurements of our mental well-being paint a concerning picture. Today, 20 percent of U.S. adults report symptoms of depression or anxiety—double the number who reported suffering from these mental health concerns in 2019. Only one in three U.S. adults now describe their mental health as "excellent"—down 28 percent from just two decades ago, and the lowest number ever reported. And in 2024, the Gallup World Poll uncovered "a dramatic decline in happiness and self-reported well-being among young adults aged 30 and below in the U.S."

I can't claim that unhealthy rumination lies at the heart of all this—there are other forces at hand—but I do think that our increased tendency toward dark thought spirals plays a role.

Perhaps one reason why answering these questions—of how many of us are ruminating too much and what to do about it—is so murky is that, according to Jill Newby, PhD, a psychologist at the University of New South Wales, in Sydney, Australia, nearly a third of us aren't even familiar with the term *rumination.* Even though researchers have studied for decades how it harms us, few of us who regularly spiral down into excessive, distressing, uncontrollable story-spinning know what *rumination* means, much less how to identify and modify its viselike hold. There is, Newby found, precious little "psychoeducation" around the vague concept of rumination.

It's hard to solve a problem you've never named and can't define. That said, even defining it can be a challenge. In the early literature on the ill effects of rumination, researchers distinguished between *worry* and *rumination.* Worry and rumination were both negative, repetitive, and chronic actions of the mind; but *worry* was defined as concern about potentially negative *future* events, and *rumination* was defined as repetitive thoughts about *past* negative experiences. In my interviews for this book, however, experts and interviewees rarely distinguished between the two. This makes sense to me: Our default mode network—as you'll soon learn—becomes overactivated by repetitive negative thinking. This is true whether that thinking is about the past or the future; it all blends into one distressing narrative. Therefore, in these pages, I'm focusing on the concept of rumination that emerges from our common vernacular, as reflected in any modern dictionary's definition of the word. According to *Merriam-Webster,* to ruminate means "to go over in the mind repeatedly" and "implies going over the same matter in one's thoughts again and again" with little "purposive thinking." We all know the feeling: we think obsessively about a problem or situation in a cyclical or repetitive way and can't shut our mind off or exit our racing thoughts.

Rumination has, of course, always been part of the human condition. It's part of the nuts and bolts of being alive. Everyone has had a distressing conversation with their partner, parent, friend, or child, and been unable to stop replaying it in their mind or fixating about how it went off track. Or become caught up in obsessing about why they didn't get that job, gig, or big contract they'd hoped for. Or found themselves rehashing agitated what-ifs about why they weren't invited to a social event, or why such and such person they'd hoped to hear from didn't call, text, or email them back.

You've no doubt had these kinds of experiences yourself. Perhaps you've found yourself, as I have, so lost in your wayward thoughts you keep rereading the same paragraph until fifteen minutes have passed, and you still haven't turned the page. Or you're baking cookies, but you're so caught up in replaying an interaction you had earlier that day with your child or spouse that you can't remember if you've already added that teaspoon of baking soda to the recipe. Most of us ruminate more than we want or ought to. And now, it seems, based on neuroscientists' findings, more than we used to. One little hiccup and our minds go off the deep end.

In his book *A Therapeutic Journey*, British philosopher Alain de Botton writes that "a healthy mind is an editing mind." It "manages to sieve, from thousands of stray, dramatic, disconcerting, or horrifying thoughts, those particular ideas and sensations" that we need "in order for us to direct our lives effectively." A well-functioning mind "recognizes the futility and cruelty of constantly finding fault with its own nature. . . . [It] can quieten its own buzzing preoccupations." All of this sounds like a very accurate description of the problem of rumination—and what it would be like to wrest free of it.

So how do we "edit" our ruminating minds and quiet our buzzing preoccupations? Once we are aware of this tendency to engage in this exhausting and unproductive mental activity, how do we find an escape route? Because of my own ruminative tendency, which has sometimes taken me to dark places, I was eager to explore the gnarly problem of how to proactively exit those tiresome, self-defeating thought loops before they drag us into stories that don't serve us. I was keen, too, to delve into this territory with my friends and acquaintances. Were they finding themselves caught up in mind drama too much of the time? And when they ruminated, what kinds of thoughts overtook them? Did they become pulled into ancient narratives like I did? Did they replay arduous conversations and wish they'd reacted differently, while chastising themselves for their missteps? And if so, how could we all liberate ourselves?

One comment Mark Trullinger made during our meeting kept coming to mind. After we'd talked about my ruminative tendencies and my desire to escape them, he'd explained, "Generally, when we talk about getting stuck in rumination, we talk about *spiraling down.* When we talk about exiting rumination, we talk about *spiraling up.*"

This is not the moment in history, I thought as he spoke, when we should let our minds slip and spiral down one iota further into darker feelings. We've never needed skills to exit rumination more than we do right now, when the whole world feels as if it's descending into anger, isolation, and resentment.

This idea—to spiral up—felt like a helpful North Star for me as I embarked on this endeavor. Instead of drowning in the torrent of my relentless thought streams each time I felt jarred by the vicissitudes of life, I wanted to learn how to spiral up and out of those dangerous waters. If I could redirect and free up my brain in this way, might that allow me more moments to experience the upside of rumination—that open-mind state in which I feel able to access inner wisdom, constructive thoughts, and a deeper well of creativity?

I was ready to spiral up toward that North Star, ready to learn how to do it.

TWO

Why We Ruminate—and the Price We Pay

ONE OF THE early pioneers in the field of psychology to study the effects of rumination on our well-being was Susan Nolen-Hoeksema, who wanted to understand why we're so prone to getting caught up in our negative mind drama in the first place. Nolen-Hoeksema found we fall into the sticky trap of rumination because we're trying to process complex emotions about the difficult things that have happened to us in the past, and to manage our fears of what might happen to us next. Our minds dangle before us the elusive promise that if we just keep rehashing our problems and replaying our fears, if we just think a little longer and a little harder, we'll find some perfect solution. Rumination gives us the illusion of working toward a solution or regaining control—engaging in what some psychologists call *effortful control* of our problems. This seductive albeit false promise—that we'll come up with answers that will make us less powerless, afraid, and alone—plunges us into a cycle of overthinking that is very hard to escape.

Although what Nolen-Hoeksema became known for was

her work on the ill effects of a ruminating mind on mental health, it's interesting to know that she came from an intellectual background that was in some ways the very opposite. She studied for her PhD at the University of Pennsylvania under the tutelage of Martin Seligman. Seligman was (and still is) widely known for studying the extensive health benefits of optimism and a positive mindset. Optimists who hold a positive outlook, Seligman found in his decades of research, are unwavering in their belief that they are worthy, capable people. When bad things happen, they know in their bones that everything will eventually come out okay. To state this in more clinical terms, Seligman defined optimism as reacting to problems with a sense of confidence; believing negative events are temporary; and knowing you have the ability to manage whatever problems arise. Optimists, he wrote, are "confronted with the same hard knocks of this world," and yet they keep a firm belief in a positive future. They don't view setbacks as a sign that they are lacking or unworthy; instead, they assume "circumstances, bad luck, or other people" brought them about. Confronted by a bad situation, optimists greet it "as a challenge and try harder."

Conversely, when those with a more negative mindset, or what I now think of as the growing contingency of ruminators among us, meet up with life's hard knocks, we're more likely to feel knocked over by them. We have trouble believing that everything will be okay. That we will be okay. When we face difficult situations or personal setbacks, pessimists/ruminators struggle to believe we are worthy beings deserving of love, care, and reassurance, including the kind of care we give ourselves. Or, as Seligman puts it, pessimists "believe bad events will last a long time, will undermine everything they do, and are their own fault." It's that last part—that we are at fault—that often feels the most abysmal.

Nolen-Hoeksema wanted to examine the flip side of a positive outlook. She was interested in what made individuals vulnerable to negative moods and, specifically, how our human tendency to get caught up in a state of rumination might influence the tenor of our mental health. She described rumination as "endless torrents of negative thoughts and emotions" that focus your attention on the causes of your distress and fears of what might happen next. Your brain becomes so caught up with agitating storytelling, it can't shift into healthy, active problem-solving. Often, Nolen-Hoeksema found, cycles of ruminating thoughts could be triggered by something as fleeting as a sarcastic remark from a partner or friend, or a feeling of being dismissed or ignored by the people we love or with whom we interact in our daily lives.

More recently, neuroscientists have found this isn't a bug in the system; rather it's a feature built into your brain. Overthinking is a survival response designed to keep you out of danger. Your brain is, first and foremost, a detective that never rests. The brain cares most about one question: "Am I safe or not safe?" Every second of your life, your brain is dancing with cues and messages from your environment—the people, places, events, and interactions that make up your life.

Of all the dangers you can face, social-emotional slights are clocked by the brain as being the most concerning. This is rooted in our evolutionary past, when social acceptance dramatically affected chances of survival. It wasn't just the bear lurking in the forest that you needed to worry about. Being excluded, slighted, left out—even just having people roll their eyes at you across the communal fire—was a portent of all kinds of possible dangers. If you were ostracized and left on your own without the support of your community, you were much more likely to face starvation, illness, or injury—or an attack from that bear. Therefore, when your mind and body pick up on signals that make you feel unsafe, rumination sets in as your brain's misguided way to resolve that sense of unsafety. Mind drama—who said or did what, how wrong it was, how wronged you were, how you should have responded differently—sets in.

Rumination can feel like dog-paddling, where your mind keeps frantically moving but going nowhere, preventing you from ever reaching your destination: the clarity and wisdom of your deepest self. As your brain revs up with ever-more-troubling thoughts, you're trying to relieve your fears, while actually intensifying them.

In William Shakespeare's comedy *As You Like It*, the young Rosalind asks the nobleman Jacques to explain his constant moodiness. Jacques replies: "It is a melancholy of mine own . . . in which my often rumination, wraps me in the most humorous sadness." Shakespeare (as was so often the case) was onto something profound five hundred years ago: A mind lost in rumination is by nature a miserable, melancholy one.

Russian novelist Fyodor Dostoevsky also understood rumination and the price we pay for it. In his 1864 book *Notes from Underground*, the narrator opines, "I swear to you that to think too much is a disease, an actual disease." The constant analysis of our own actions and those of others leads to what Dostoevsky terms a "furious dissatisfaction" that hampers our ability to form meaningful connections with other people. It also corrodes our sense of self.

In other words, the more you ruminate, the more likely you are to turn on yourself with derision. And the longer you stay snared in these negative loops of self-talk, the more likely they are to lead to depression. Left unchecked, a routinely ruminating mind is, Nolen-Hoeksema found in the clinical studies she conducted, one of the biggest predictors of anxiety, depression, substance abuse, and eating disorders.

Following up on Nolen-Hoeksema's research after her death in 2013, neuroscientists were able to reveal the exact location where rumination activity takes place in our brains' gray matter—in the default mode network, the area that had appeared overactive and illuminated in red in my own brain scans—and also to use brain scans to predict the possible effects of rumination on our future health.

In a 2023 study using fMRI, Dartmouth and Johns Hopkins neuroscientists found that individuals whose brains frequently repeat this neural pattern are significantly more likely to develop major depressive disorder—often quickly, within the next year. (One more reason to explore how to escape our mind drama. None of us wants this habit to become a slippery slope into something more troubling.) Other studies have shown that rumination is also predictive of cognitive decline. (No one wants that, either.) And researchers who study Alzheimer's disease are now targeting the default mode network for treatments; in patients with Alzheimer's, brain activity in the default mode network, which plays a role in memory and cognition, becomes notably altered.

Other researchers have found that rumination is linked to a much higher risk of stress-related physical conditions, including heart disease, high blood pressure, chronic pain, and irritable bowel syndrome. The degree of our tendency to ruminate even predicts how well we'll heal after surgery; brooding and ruminating predict poorer clinical outcomes and a longer period of recovery.

How much we brood and ruminate also shapes the tenor of our relationships. When we spend time lost in our mind drama, we embellish feelings not just of self-contempt but of contempt for others. Many of the ill-chosen words and deeds we later regret emerge from stuck-in-our-head recursive thinking, marinating in memories of what others said or did to us or failed to say or do. When we attack others in some irrational or disproportionate way or turn on ourselves with shame or self-loathing, it's often our untamed ruminations that are to blame. When we're lost in rumination, we're also more likely to lose track of appointments, where we put things, what we need to buy when we go to the store, and the details of our daily lives. (Just ask my dog Winnie!)

And now, thanks to the hours we spend scrolling social media and clicking on things that outrage us or make us feel inferior, anxious about the future, or left out (FOMO is so often a social-media-fueled phenomenon), we become further trapped in this toxic state. Taken together, all these outcomes of rumination, according to the experts who study this mental act, make it one of the most corrosive habits we can engage in when it comes to our health, draining us perhaps more than any other single activity.

Many, if not most, of us are feeling this. In a 2022 nationwide study by the American Psychological Association, nearly three-quarters of adults reported either "worrying constantly," "feeling overwhelmed," or experiencing negative "changes in sleeping habits." Among youth ages eighteen to thirty-four, the majority say they're so distracted by stressful, negative thought loops that it's hard to focus or function. In a study released in 2025 by the Global Mind Project, which uses the Mind Health Quotient to study the well-being of one million people across the globe, today's "sharp decline" in youth mental health is marked by growing challenges with "cognitive functions, such as planning and focus," and "emotional regulation." Among high school students, stress is driving extraordinary levels of despair; in a 2023 study from the Centers for Disease Control and Prevention (CDC), 57 percent of teen girls reported feeling "persistently sad or hopeless."

Much of this can be traced, as we know, to the social and emotional landscape in which youth are forming their early sense of themselves. Young people are experiencing an unprecedented scale of rejection across social media apps, online platforms, group chats, dating apps, and the college process—more rejections in a week than most of us who are now adults faced in a year. It's little wonder that in surveys of twelfth graders, teens are more likely, compared to twenty-five years ago, to become lost in what's known as *self-derogation*—judging themselves in a diminishing way, as in "I feel I do not have much to be proud of," "I feel I can't do anything right," and "Sometimes I think I'm no good at all."

These are all expressions of pure rumination.

I've seen this distress writ large across the country over the past five years. In one of my workshop series, my Post-it Note Project, I go into schools to work with students. One of the many exercises I do with them is to ask them to write down for me, anonymously, what they wish they could tell the adults in their lives but can't. When they pass their Post-it notes to me and I read them aloud, one after the other, the room goes silent. It's so ubiquitous—the perseverative nature of their negative, cyclical thoughts—it hurts all of us to hear it: "It feels like my whole life is made of mistakes." "I can't stop thinking about everything I've done wrong." "I am a burden." "I have to be perfect." "Ninety percent of the time, I smile, but I'm not happy." "The future only holds more stress; it will never end." "Everything is not okay!" "Ask me if I'm really fine!" "You don't know how hard it is to compare yourself to everyone 24-7." I could go on. Interestingly, as dire as all these statements are, as painful as they are to listen to, there is often a palpable feeling of relief afterward, as the students realize that others share their feelings.

What strikes me is that no matter what age group I'm working with, this feeling of relief always emerges once people learn that they're not the only ones ruminating, the only ones to feel this pain. Knowing, finally, that they are *not* alone is healing in and of itself. My guess is that the degree of relief people feel at revealing this proclivity to ruminate is in proportion to the fear and shame they carry about it.

It's a double whammy: We're spending more time ruminating than ever, but we're also so embarrassed by it, shamed by it, we can't talk about it—which means we can't get the support we need. Professor Susan David, PhD, a psychologist at Harvard Medical School, found in a study of seventy thousand people that one-third of us "either judge ourselves for having so-called bad emotions, like sadness, anger or even grief . . . or actively try to push aside these feelings." As a culture, we also judge others for having difficult negative thoughts and emotions, viewing them as a character weakness, a flaw.

Knowing that rumination is a propensity shared by many others is beneficial—but those of us who engage in this mental habit need a lot more help than that, and the good news is that neuroscientists have been investigating new ways to stop our ruminating thoughts and opt out of this destructive habit.

During a recent lecture at a medical school, I discussed some of the science I was learning about the ill consequences of excessive rumination. Following my talk, a young man, whom I'll call Sam, approached me. His brown eyes were rimmed red with exhaustion. As he talked, he fidgeted with a pen, tapping it against his hand as if signaling the Morse code for anxiety. Sam knew enough about neuroscience to understand that his habit of rumination has probably had a bad effect on his mental and physical well-being, but he was skeptical about what science could teach him about how to stop it. In fact, learning how detrimental rumination is only made him feel worse about his "spinning out" thoughts, because he finds it "impossible *not* to go there."

On the day we met, Sam was churning over something a medical school professor, who was also his adviser, had said to him earlier that week. "He told me that after all the interest he's shown in me and his belief in my potential, it was 'unseemly' for me not to have selected surgery—his specialty—as my own," Sam recounted. "He wants me to follow in his footsteps, but I don't feel ready to make that choice."

I ask Sam to take me inside his torrents of thoughts. "What does it sound like inside your head when you replay that interaction?"

Sam winces as if it's all too unpleasant to bear (or bare), before sharing: "I worry about what he's going to say to the rest of the faculty about me behind my back. He is that kind of prof who likes to trash people when they're not around. Is he going to trash me? Maybe I should just leave med school; it's not what I thought it was going to be. It's not really about helping people; it's an ego race. But if I left, I would still have these fucking crushing loans to pay. And if I stay, how am I going to make a living? I've got so much debt! I'll never have a life. I'm never going to meet the right person, I don't have time, and dating apps are a soul suck, and even if I did meet someone, I'll never be able to afford to start a family or buy a house." Sam pauses and catches his breath. "I just see this past in which all I've done is make the wrong decisions—maybe going to med school was a mistake?—and this future in which I'm stressed and broke and alone."

I ask Sam, who is growing tenser with every word, what

this feels like in his body. "Like I'm being squeezed by a boa constrictor. When I try to pry it off, it grips tighter." He pauses. "Sometimes, I'll be sitting with a patient, and I'm not even there; I'm immobilized in my head. And then I feel like a fraud, like, here they are, hoping I can help them, and I'm letting them down, the way I let everyone down, and the whole cycle starts over again."

I tell Sam that in my research, I've found there are science-based, accessible ways to stave off and exit our ruminations. That said, I emphasize, the goal isn't to hammer them down—doing so will only make them stronger—but to listen to them so we can see what they have to tell us. I tell Sam that, if he is interested in going on this journey, I think I can help him develop a skill set that will simultaneously keep him from getting sucked into and hypnotized by his storylines, while also shedding light on them. What I've found is this: By decoding our personal habits of rumination, we can access insights into our life stories that we might not be able to gain any other way. And these insights can lead us to a new, intimate understanding of ourselves that touches into every area of our lives.

Sam's eyes brighten a bit as I tell him this, as if registering hope about the possibility of change. Our conversation marked the beginning of a journey that unfolded over many months—a time when I offered Sam the same gentle strategies, thoughtful techniques, and practical tips that I'll be sharing with you. Some ideas spoke to him more deeply than others, as I imagine will be true for you. Still, I believe each one has its own quiet value, worthy of your reflection and consideration. I hope you'll approach them with curiosity and openness, and discover which ones resonate most with your own inner life.

THREE

A Hidden Desire Behind Our Mind Drama

The Longing to Belong

I KNOW MY friend Virginia to be full of life, creative, brilliant. For years, she's helped run a prestigious Washington, D.C., think tank. But I also happen to know she finds herself caught up in brooding rumination far too often. I know this because much of our twenty-year friendship has revolved around talking each other "off the ledge" from what we call our "perseverations." When I tell Virginia what I'm investigating, she immediately relates, admitting she's recently found herself caught in her head even more than she used to be, "returning again and again to conversations and feelings that were hurtful and full of self-loathing—but without any resolution." Recently, in her late forties, she's turned her hand to painting and has started to win some small recognition. But her tendency to get caught up in negative thoughts about her work is getting in the way of finding her voice in her art.

"Yesterday, I was sitting in a painting workshop that involved critiquing one another's work. People were a lot harder on me than I was on them. My mind fell into a hole, where I rehashed other people's comments and critiques. I was up half the night, replaying the whole thing. It felt a lot like times at work when I've been left out during important conversations and my boss would go to someone else for advice while ignoring my input." Virginia's brow furrowed, a sigh escaping her lips. Despite her mental exhaustion, she was dressed in her usual artsy style: a green shawl draped over her shoulders; blue, wide-legged trousers; her thick, copper hair pinned up neatly with a silver hairpin at the back of her head. She was holding herself together, the way people do when they're worn-out, even when no one is watching. "If I let them, these small injuries can become excruciating, consuming me. And when I'm in that headspace, I can't forgive people for not seeing my worth. My brain perseverates on things like, *Wait, does my work suck? Was I being difficult when I critiqued them? Why did he come down so hard on me? What gives her the right to be so critical? Her work isn't so great. Why is he listening to my coworker and not to what I have to say?* And then I feel so ashamed of what I'm thinking, like I'm a shithead because I'm so ungenerous. Then I'm doubly pissed off because, wow, now I'm letting something small that happened days or weeks ago ruin so many hours of my life. It's so painful. Especially because in those moments it feels as if I don't matter to the people who matter to me."

In our era of disconnection, when we so often find ourselves scrolling for belonging online versus in real life, it can be easy to overlook this visceral need for what Virginia very insightfully calls "mattering." In the 1940s, American psychologist Abraham Harold Maslow first put forth his famous theory of psychological well-being, in which he argued that unless our most pressing human needs are filled, we cannot realize our full potential. Having defined those needs in a hierarchy of their importance, Maslow deemed the most basic needs to be for food, shelter, and water. But second only to your body's instinctual survival needs is your longing for belonging; to feel loved, valued, and cherished by the people with whom you share your life—the family that raised you, the partners, parents, children, colleagues, and friends with whom you spend your waking hours. Next in Maslow's hierarchy is the need to know that others in your life hold you in esteem and think well of you. You are respected. If you can satisfy these first three tiers, you're well positioned to discover your unique abilities, rise into your full potential, and contribute your gifts to the wider world. But if you are deprived of any of these three primary human tiers, all your mental and emotional energy will go to trying to meet them, and you will not have the energy you need to fulfill yourself.

When Virginia talks about feeling like she doesn't matter, and how this feeling plunges her into rumination, I can't help but wonder how this might also be hindering her ability to become the artist she longs to become.

How Our Early Stories Shape Our Mind Drama

It's our earliest relationships that program our default mode network for how well we will be able to respond to slights and disappointments, conflict and rejection, and the deeper losses we will all experience at one time or another in our lives. This is why it's so important for our first caregivers to make us feel cherished and valued. The messages they send to us about ourselves are crucial to developing a sense of self-worth and have immense implications for our lifelong well-being.

So much of our unhealthy rumination is rooted in unprocessed emotions from these early relationships. The default mode network is where we first absorb the message that we matter, or we don't. This begins in the womb, but it's outside the womb that the default mode network gets wired up fast, as it responds to face-to-face interactions with our first caregivers, and the degree to which those interactions cause us to feel safe, versus in some kind of danger. Before we even have language, we take in this message of mattering through our parents' touch and tone of voice, and later, their words.

At the Institute for Early Life Adversity Research at Dell Medical School at the University of Texas at Austin, psychologist Elizabeth Lippard, PhD, reviewed hundreds of studies on the consequences of different types of early life adversity and zeroed in on the two types of childhood experiences that stood out as being particularly likely to engender adult anxiety and depression:

1. Being emotionally or verbally humiliated, as in put down, made fun of, or routinely criticized by a parent or caregiver (also known as *emotional abuse*).
2. Being ignored, made to feel neglected, feeling that no one in your family looked out for you, had your back, or cared about you in a way that let you know you mattered, you belonged (also known as *emotional neglect*).*

It might be tempting to think these childhood experiences are rare—or, one might hope, rarer than they were during cultural periods when popular parenting styles were more authoritarian and disciplinary-driven. But research shows that's far from the case. Even amid the seemingly self-esteem-attuned cultural approach to "gentle parenting" today, kids report feeling quashed and demoralized by the weight of parental expectations and slights. In a first-of-its-kind study, the CDC asked teens to self-report the adversities they faced and to examine how those adversities affected them. In its 2024 report, it found that not only are high schoolers today experiencing higher levels of adversity, but the most common source of adversity they face is at home. Sixty-one percent of teens said they experience being put down or insulted by a parent or adult at home. Sixty-five percent of teens said that the adversity they faced often led to "sadness and hopelessness." Will these kids be more likely to grow up to be future ruminators? You can probably answer that question for yourself.

Researchers who study the adolescent brain have indeed found, when comparing brain images of adolescents who struggle with depression to those who do not, that teens with

* Other researchers have found that, not surprisingly, sexual abuse is also more likely to engender later mental health concerns.

depression show an overactive default mode network. They are spending great swaths of time in rumination.

There is no one better to turn to for help understanding why these experiences of early adversity predispose us to more frequent rumination later in life than Ruth Lanius, MD, PhD, who is professor of psychiatry and the Harris-Woodman Chair in Mind-Body Medicine at Western University of Canada, where she is the director of the Clinical Research Program for PTSD. Lanius began her training thirty years ago, and she took her time exploring the many and diverse areas that interested her, which is why she has degrees in two different fields—and is able to draw on research that comes from so many different disciplines.

As Lanius explained to me when I talked to her about the impact of early life adversity, "Routine emotional rejection, feeling criticized or abandoned or unseen by a caregiver, alters the development of a child's default mode network, and their sense of self, because it elicits an immediate burst of stratospheric rumination as the brain tries to process that the person who is supposed to care for you isn't going to do that." This is why changes in the default mode network that begin in childhood—as they so often do—can require concerted effort to undo. (And yet, as you will see, it is very possible to undo these changes, once you have a neuroscience-based road map to guide you.) It is also why we so rarely forget the things our parents or caregivers said or did that hurt us, and why circumstances that bring to mind old, familiar wounds still set off reverberations decades later—or forever. Your ruminations are regurgitating the same emotions, fears, and sense of helplessness you felt when you were very young.

This echoes findings by Susan Nolen-Hoeksema that showed that ruminating about how a recent scenario in which you felt left out, dismissed, or hurt can prompt the recall of other, similar negative autobiographical memories. These memories and montages arise in our minds, unbidden, not just because the feelings they engender are painful in and of themselves but because they feel all too familiar.

We are, to quote the poet Adrienne Rich, "root-tangled in the grit of human arrangements and relationships: how we are with each other." That entanglement showed up in Jill Newby's survey of nearly two hundred people, which found that the most common trigger for rumination is challenging conversations and exchanges in close relationships or social interactions. *People* are the biggest complication that life throws our way. This makes me think of the Apple TV series *Severance*, in which people volunteer to undergo a procedure in which their consciousness is split between who they are in their personal lives (their "outies") and who they are at work (their "innies"). They choose this bifurcated life because they desperately long for a daily eight-hour break from perseverating about what pains them in their personal lives, almost all of which stems from their losses, their longings, in their relationships.

What wounded us when we were young echoes within us still. These moments that influence or recur in our adult ruminations might emerge as flashes of emotions, or as small flickers of memory, like images in a slideshow, of scenes of humiliation or hurt. You were five and accidentally stepped on flowers in the garden while playing with a friend, and your mom raged at you. Or you were six and struggling to tie your shoes when your dad snapped, "What's wrong with you?" You were eight and struggling to figure out a math problem, and your mother barked, "You're such a dunce!" You were ten and missed the goal when playing soccer, and the whole way home, your father wouldn't speak to you. You were eleven and trying on a bathing suit when your mom pinched your waist and said, "Look at that roll. You're getting chubby!" You were thirteen and came home upset about how your two best friends were making fun of you, and your mom asked, "What did you do to them?" and your dad told you, "Toughen up!" And so on.

In looking back on difficult moments in your own childhood, you may be inclined to dismiss them as too minor to be a problem in your adult life (despite the fact that you can still remember them so vividly all these years later). We often assume trauma is defined as beatings from an alcoholic father, or a mother who locked you in the closet, but researchers who study the effects of childhood adversity on well-being have shown that trauma often shows up much more quietly in a child's home. Parents might be physically present, but they're so preoccupied with their own struggles, or haven't yet healed from their own invisible wounds, that they can't tend to your pain or shore you up when you need it most. Or maybe they tried, valiantly, to offer you what love they could, but life had drained or broken them, for reasons you were too young to understand at the time. This kind of childhood loss is subtle, almost ordinary, and yet it leaves its mark.

Even if you don't have anything blatantly traumatic in your past, you, too, may be hurting. There is a reason why, at the time, the experiences you can't forget struck deep. Whatever happened to you, your hurt is warranted. These internalized hurts often whisper to us for a lifetime, starting when we are very young. This is why when children are alone and engaging in pretend play with dolls, stuffed animals, or action figures, they often repeat things their parents said to them. A girl whose mother scolded her, in a moment of exasperation, "Jane, you ask so many questions, you're wearing on my last nerve!" might scold her teddy bear with the same words later that day. She's trying to school herself not to behave in a way that will irritate her mother. Jane assumes her mother's words are not only true but are a core part of her identity. *I am a person who wears on people's nerves.* In this way, your experiences in childhood shape your belief about your self-worth.

As Lanius explains, "The child brain has to find a way to deal with the impossible—that as a child, you don't matter to your caregiver. The brain needs a story, a reason why this is happening. If it can come up with a plausible narrative for why your parent is behaving this way—a self-blaming one—maybe you can adjust how you behave so you finally get your needs met."

The power of these moments and events from childhood make them so "sticky" that they may arise again and again in our heads, often against our will. (I use the word *sticky* here because once these memories materialize, they prove hard to shake off.)

For me, the stickiest of all are the memories of my father's death when I was twelve, and of everything that happened after. My father went into the hospital for minor surgery—he'd be there for just a few days, everyone told me—and I never saw him again. As I learned later—much later—the surgeon neglected to read my father's list of medications, which included a recent course of cortisone. He was sewn up with sutures known to dissolve in steroids like cortisone. After the surgery, his sutures opened. He had internal hemorrhaging that went undiagnosed until he developed sepsis and died. On my thirteenth birthday, a few days after his death, my mother gave me a gold locket he'd preordered for my birthday from our local jeweler. On the front were my initials. After I opened the box, I pulled the locket out and let the gold chain dangle on my fingers. When I flipped it over, I saw that on the back it read, "To Donna, Love Daddy." Those were the last words I ever heard from my father.

His loss radiated across all areas of my life. My mother's descent into an intractable (and entirely understandable) depression made it feel as if I had lost two parents in one fell swoop. Our extended family imploded. Relatives took my father's death as an opportunity to wrest control of the family business away from my mother, leaving her, and us, to fend for ourselves. My childhood forever in the rearview mirror, I took on as many odd jobs over the next years as I could—shelving books at the library, busing tables at an Italian restaurant, working in a crab house—to relieve any burden on my mother for my own upkeep, while stuffing down my emotions, never speaking to anyone about what it felt like to lose the one person I'd felt certain had really loved and known—and wanted to know—me. Unfathomable, unspoken loss; my mother's disappearance into a fog of anguish, hopelessness, and dejection. The acts of betrayal by people we'd trusted became the defining aspects of my childhood and continued to resonate for many years into my adult life.

◆ ◆ ◆ ◆

The death of a parent is a serious wound, but there are so many others. Perhaps, for you, it was a parent who was cruel with their words or deeds, or failed to support you when siblings or peers bullied you. Or parents who fought bitterly but stayed together, so that growing up in that family was like navigating an emotional war zone. Or perhaps there was simply no adult to whom you could turn when you needed someone to tell you that everything would be okay when your friend group turned on you in high school. Whoever or whatever hurt you, these feelings were encoded into the neural structure of your default mode network.

The default mode network desperately wants to help you with this—it's just not very good at it because its wiring is laid down so early that it's hard to change it. So, as children, we tell ourselves the story that what's happening to us must be our fault. *I'm a burden. I ruin things. I don't deserve love. Something's wrong with me. My body is ugly and wrong. I did something wrong.* Such beliefs take hold early on, when we are too young to question their validity, and they tend to stick around.

It's hard to forget the things that hurt us.

In one 2022 study, researchers had over two hundred young people fill out a questionnaire about their experiences of childhood adversity. Participants reported varying levels—some had a lot, others little. Investigators then used brain imaging to quantify activity in all the participants' default mode networks, as well as the degree of connectivity across the whole brain. They found significant relationships between individuals' experiences and degrees of early life adversity and "dysregulated connectivity" in their default mode networks—which correlated to their emotional states and their behavior.

When the pain of your early stories and beliefs are triggered in your adult life, "the default mode network gets dysregulated, just as it did when those wounds first occurred," Lanius explained. "Our brains are wired to repeat what is familiar, think the same thoughts, feel the same emotions, and have the same reactions that formed us when we were young." When we're raised with negative conditioning—criticism, belittling, neglect of our emotional needs—we later regurgitate this response in the way we talk to ourselves.

You might think that by being hard on yourself, or self-punitive, you'll be motivated to change in a positive way to escape the self-criticism, but the brain doesn't work that way. All that happens, regardless of any temporary, superficial changes in behavior you might make, is that you create even deeper neural grooves in your default mode network, which show up as self-flagellation, self-doubt, and self-silencing, further eroding your faith in who you are.

Chronic childhood stress and uncertainty change the brain in myriad ways—not just in the default mode network. Adversity in childhood alters neural connectivity in other crucial brain areas, including the amygdala, the danger and alarm center of your brain; the hippocampus, where you process memories and emotions; and the prefrontal cortex, your brain's decision-making and control center.

The changes that happen inside each brain region influence every other area, rippling out across your neurobiology. As the default mode network doubles down on regurgitating old stories and self-beliefs, it further disconnects from the rest of your thinking, feeling brain. It's firing at full speed—but it quickly becomes a closed circuit on a locked loop. "It can't interface with the rest of your brain in the way a healthy, integrated brain should," Lanius adds. She attributes the disconnection between the default network and the thinking brain to input from what she terms your *survival brain.* The survival brain, which includes your brain stem, cerebellum, and midbrain, sits at the lower back of your skull. It is deeply affected by childhood adversity in ways that—throughout your life—can quickly spike your default mode network into rumination. Lanius breaks this down in a way I find very useful: "In the aftermath of adversity, your survival brain becomes poised to react to new sources of danger. Each time your survival brain senses a threat, it uploads raw, incoming sensory information—pure, unfiltered emotion, arousal, and fear—to the rest of your brain. The closer you sense danger is, the more you freeze, and your thinking brain shuts down."

But here's the thing: All of this is happening beneath your conscious awareness. And what's under there is always the overarching fear that it is our unlovability, our utter invisibility, our not mattering, that has brought us here, into this moment. So we talk to ourselves in ways that make us feel small. In adult life, this shows up as feeling that any problem with our children means we're inherently not good enough as a parent, that any struggles we have with a project at work mean we're not as efficient as our colleagues, that any snide comment directed our way is worth listening to.

One moment of feeling dismissed or denigrated and we're sliding down that slippery slope into a world of negative self-beliefs. Like Virginia, we fear we truly are flawed and unlovable; that we really don't matter to the people to whom we long to matter, including ourselves. The lack of mattering is a lack that always hurts.

But we didn't come into the world this way, convinced of our personal worthlessness, always certain we're falling short, convinced we should be different or better than we are. We are conditioned by our caregivers, who were undoubtedly conditioned by *their* caregivers to believe they, too, were unworthy, and never learned the skills to break this neurobiological inheritance.

Perhaps the worst part is that this flinch reaction, to turn on ourselves, feels so instinctive that we automatically believe our self-defeating thoughts are true.

This idea—that our patterns for rumination become honed in childhood—isn't theoretical. Consider a 2023 study in which researchers from the United Kingdom, the United States, and

Germany studied 183 children ages twelve and younger. Half had a history of adversity, including emotional neglect and emotional abuse; half did not. Researchers gave all the children mental tasks, then observed and questioned them to see if, under the stress of completing those tasks, their minds wandered in ruminative ways ("Were you thinking about the task or something else?"). They then scanned children's brains using MRI. They found that even with minimal provocation, children with a history of adversity showed alterations in areas of the brain associated with brooding and fretting, or what the researchers called *spontaneous rumination thought patterns.* These children were more likely to become caught in a snare of past-oriented negative thoughts, had fewer positive thoughts, and were less able to conjure hopeful scenarios about their futures. Researchers concluded that children who face chronic adversity develop overactive neural networks that trigger rapid-fire ruminative thoughts. This, over time, creates the "neurobiological coordinates," or neural patterns, that can manifest as clinical depression.

In a separate study of nearly six hundred American college students, those who experienced childhood adversity, including emotional neglect and abuse, physical neglect and abuse, and sexual abuse, were significantly more likely to ruminate and, not surprisingly, experience higher levels of "psychological stress while attending college."

Nolen-Hoeksema found similar evidence of the association between adversity and rumination, and also observed the tendency for rumination on one topic to spark a "global, repetitive, self-focused style" of rumination about other issues in one's life. I certainly recognize this globalizing tendency in my life. I'll be thinking about something I said and wish I could retract, or remembering with mortification how I'd stumbled on the jumble of computer wires on the floor as I walked onto a lecture stage before giving a talk—and suddenly my mind is off and running. I'll think of the person who hasn't responded to an email—*Have I done something wrong there, too?* Next thing I know, my mind skitters to the prickly thing a colleague said to me. *Why is she always so critical, so undermining?* If this sequence goes on long enough, I'll start to chastise myself for my health issues, which have been serious over the years, blaming myself for the emotional and financial cost they've wreaked on my family. Suddenly, it feels as if everything I'm doing, saying, being, is all wrong. *I* am all wrong.

This tendency, Mark Trullinger had explained when we reviewed my brain scans, was writ large in my neural circuitry: "I can see by the activity in your default mode network that your neural pattern for rumination was set in motion when you were a child, when you encountered some kind of significant adversity. And that's been exacerbated by emotional and physical ordeals you've faced in your adult life." More tea leaves, which had amazed me.

After the devastating loss of my father, I often found myself—far more often than I understood at the time—lost in my own head, ruminating, trying yet failing to process the many losses and traumas that now defined my life. But I rarely spoke of any of what I felt, because who would I have talked to? My father, who was always the person I had turned to in the past, was gone, my mother was heroically struggling to keep herself and her four kids afloat. I fell silent. So silent that other kids nicknamed me, in the parlance of the day, a real *space cadet*, as if I were in training for a lifetime of getting lost in my own thoughts. We'd be sitting in eighth-grade French class, and suddenly another student would poke me in the arm with their pencil eraser: "Where are you? *Earth to Donna!*"

Meanwhile, my mother, grief-stricken and terrified about what the future might hold, was simply unreachable to me. In high school, it was a teacher who noticed that no one seemed to have taken much interest in my academic future and took it upon herself to take me on a college tour. One of my older brothers helped me fill out college applications. The librarians at the library where I worked after school helped me file for scholarships. All these things happened more or less beneath my mother's radar. If others hadn't stepped in, I might never have made it to college.

But I hadn't always been such a space cadet. Before my father's death, I had been a confident, even loquacious, twelve-year-old. My sixth-grade teacher had once taken me aside to ask if I would befriend a girl new to our class. "If you do, everyone will follow," he'd said. "You're a natural leader." But by the time I entered seventh grade, my father having died two weeks earlier, I'd gone selectively mute. One day at school, in the fall after his death, I stood up to give a book report in my history class, but no words would come out of my mouth. I stood there, peering down at my index cards, confident about my research, my ideas, and what I'd written down, perhaps even imagining that by being a good history student, a stellar reporter, I might do something to honor the memory of my father, the newspaper editor. But hard as I tried to speak, nothing came, not a squeak. "That's okay, Donna. You can sit down," my teacher said, compassion in his eyes.

I still remember that small moment of being seen, of my feelings mattering to someone, of feeling that I mattered, precisely because in those years following my father's death, it was such an infrequent experience. (A shout-out to you, Mr. Zimmerman, wherever you are.)

But what if we each had a bespoke road back to heal our wounds, and that road could be traveled by listening to what our ruminations are trying to tell us? What if our ruminations are encoded with messages that can lead us back home to heal our wounded selves?

Imagine if you could examine your ruminations to recognize how your wounds are still influencing you, and by achieving that clarity, move past them. How might this change how you deal with adversity in the future? How different could your life be if it weren't dominated by these endless internal conversations about how unworthy you are? How freeing would it be, and how much energy would that give you to access more of your internal wisdom, and more of your innate creativity?

The good news is we need not keep breaking our own hearts, feeling we do not belong, that we were never lovable or never will be. The neural structure of the default mode network remains plastic throughout your life. There are techniques and strategies that can rewire it, no matter your story, your wounds, or your age. (As you'll read later, Ruth Lanius even showed me the results of a new mind-body-based treatment that in only eight sessions can create profound changes in how we think and feel, helping to deliver us from early trauma.)

In what follows, you'll be learning about everything I have learned about these strategies, which I hope will help you better understand your inner world and move closer to living the life you truly desire—and deserve to revel in.

II

What Are Your Ruminations Trying to Tell You?

FOUR

Seeing Through Your Mind Drama

Differentiate Between Helpful Thinking and Unhelpful Overthinking

ONE OF MY neighborhood friends, whom I'll call Paola, is in what I have always thought to be a uniquely simpatico partnership. She and her husband, Will, are in their late fifties. They work for the same international aid foundation and travel the globe helping to get food, medicine, and vaccines into wherever people in the world are in need. They are good people. When they're home, they cook, hike, garden, and run errands together. They enjoy the same TV shows, root for the same sports teams, and always seem to be laughing. I think of them as inseparable.

But one afternoon, while I was out on a walk, I ran into Paola. Surprised to see her out walking alone, I asked, "Where's Will?"

She gestured, throwing her thumb back over her shoulder toward her driveway. Will stood near their trash cans, hands on hips, too far away from us to hear our conversation. "He's back there being a big jerk!" Paola said.

I laughed and said, "Really?" I told her how I always admired their effortless togetherness, how playful they were together—like kids still in love.

"I do love him," Paola said. "But honestly, the things that can come out of his mouth would astonish you. He can be so asinine."

It was several weeks later before I saw Paola without Will again. We were both ducking into our local post office early one Saturday morning. She was in line ahead of me, tall, thin, wearing trekking shorts and Birkenstocks, her graying hair in a braid that hung down her back. After we greeted each other, she asked, her voice gravelly, as if the morning hadn't quite let go of her yet, if I had time for a coffee. We went to the café next door. After we sat down, Paola looked at me, her hands wrapped around a coffee mug. "I've been thinking about what I said before," she told me. "About Will. I'm sorry I vented like that." But, she added, as if by way of explanation for her outburst, "he really struggles with his verbal filter." On the one hand, he's sometimes very funny. On the other, words "come out of his mouth before he's thought them through." When he's stressed, she explained, he has an especially poor filter. He's also perpetually impatient, wanting everything to happen now, so he's always in a rush, always pushing Paola to hurry up even when there's absolutely no reason to do so. He just seems to need that sense of urgency all the time, she told me. This dynamic, when they met in their early twenties, while tiresome, did not feel hugely problematic. At fifty-nine, it did.

"Yesterday, we were getting in the car to run errands, and he started to pull the car out of the driveway before I'd even gotten my other foot in and closed the car door—my foot was still sticking out the door! I told him, 'Don't ever do that again!' " There is something in the way she says this, a kind of loneliness, maybe, or just the wish that their relationship could be easier, less fractious.

Will couldn't understand why Paola was upset. "He said, 'Oh, you know I was only joking around!' "

The problem is, Paola continues, "he's always a kid! We were kids when we met. But I'm tired. I need him to be a grown-up now."

This childishness, she goes on, was one reason why she didn't push the idea of having children when Will told her, early on, he wasn't sure he wanted to have them. She loved him but wasn't sure how he'd be as a dad, and besides, she didn't carry a burning desire to become a mother. So it was fine. But now, Paola feels . . . alone. "The other day, we were out running, and I fell and kind of twisted my ankle. It wasn't terrible, but it hurt, and he didn't even help me get up. Later that evening, I was keeping ice on the swollen area while we were watching TV. Will told me, as if it were funny, 'You'd better get better fast! We go to Zimbabwe next week; we already have the plane tickets!' "

Smart and dedicated as Will is, Paola finds herself wishing he weren't "such a gray-haired teenager. I wish he had the capacity to say, 'I'm sorry your ankle is swollen. Does it hurt? What do you need? How can I help?' But I don't think he can handle the idea of my not being super healthy and raring to go; he can't tolerate any weakness in me, and if I express any needs, he just tries to dismiss me with a joke or a put-down."

This sometimes makes Paola wonder "if I should have chosen differently." The other day, she and Will were watching an old Wes Anderson film, *Fantastic Mr. Fox*, and in the movie, after another one of Mr. Fox's misadventures, Mrs. Fox tells Mr. Fox, "I love you, too, but I shouldn't have married you." That, says Paola, "hit me. I keep hearing that play in my head. Or I imagine other scenarios of how my life might have gone. I think about the kids I might have had, kids who, by now, would be finishing college. Then I start rehashing all the times when I needed Will to be a grown-up, but he couldn't. Even after my mother died last year, he found it hard to muster the empathy I needed. When I think about the future, I wonder when I'm old and infirm, will he even be able to love me? I'm probably thinking about this more because I've had some health problems recently."

I tell Paola about the research I'm doing on rumination. When I tell her the title of this book, she chimes in, "That's me! That's me! Once I get going, it's a thought avalanche I can't stop. And I hate it." Then she pauses. "But how else do you work through things, if not by thinking about them?"

It can be hard to know the difference between when you're productively processing your emotions after stressful interactions versus stuck in rumination and mind drama. Our culture places a premium on thinking and analyzing as a sign of our intelligence. But there's thinking... and then there's overthinking. The first can yield results. The latter is a trap, preventing us from doing anything proactive about our concerns.

For this reason, it can help to have a checklist to distinguish healthy emotional processing from mind drama. (If you're still wondering if unwanted patterns of rumination and overthinking are fueling distress in your life, see the appendix, where I offer a ten-minute questionnaire to help you answer that question.) I suggest to Paola that as soon as she thinks she might be falling into overthinking, she pose the following questions to herself:

- *Does focusing on my problems feel like I'm just going round and round in circles, or does it seem as though it might lead somewhere?* According to psychologist Sally Winston, if you're not gaining a new perspective, that's a sign you're stuck in the illusion of problem-solving versus processing your emotions. Conversely, if after thinking through a negative event you're able to tap into why you feel the way you do, acknowledge your feelings, regulate your emotions, put your experience in perspective, and take constructive action, you're not ruminating, you're engaged in higher-level problem-solving.
- *Do I feel like I'm choosing to think about these things, or that I'd like to stop but can't?* Does your rumination have an end

point, or are your thoughts like a car without brakes? If you were pulled away from your thought stream to get up for a glass of water, or to get in the car to go pick up your kids, would you feel sucked right back into your ruminating thought loops afterward? Does your mind drama have its own momentum, its own "mind"? If you feel like your spinning thoughts are something that's happening to you, not something you're choosing to do, you're caught in rumination.

- *Are my mental stories familiar?* Have you heard these same refrains many times before in your head? If your mental stories are like watching film clips you've already seen, you're definitely ruminating.
- *Am I searching for a solution where there is none?* Is there any aspect of this scenario that is under your control? Anything here you can truly solve by just sitting here, rehashing it? We often think we can't solve a problem unless we focus all our mental energy on it. But if there is no resolution to the situation, this behavior just gives you a false sense of productivity. So take note of that and how much energy you put into something for which there exists no "fix." If you have that sense that you probably shouldn't be thinking about this situation anymore but can't help yourself, you're probably thinking about a situation that has no perfect solution, or a solution that is beyond your locus of control.

   Just because a problem presents itself doesn't mean you have to chase the fix. Sometimes, the most helpful thing you can do is to recognize that and stop the chasing. If it's out of your hands, why not free your mind from it, too?
- *Do I feel better after ruminating—or worse?* Yes, that's a rhetorical question. In my own experience as a veteran ruminator, I've learned that often the most helpful thing I can do when I catch myself ruminating is to ask myself a single question: *How often do I want to feel this way?* When our rumination is made up of a litany of our failings, faults,

mistakes, regrets, or other feelings of unworthiness, or a similar litany about what we perceive to be the shortcomings of others, we usually end up feeling awful. "Rumination is identified not by the content of the worry but how it acts and feels," Winston explains. Rumination just multiplies and prolongs our misery. So, if you feel tenser, agitated, and unhappy after ruminating, or your mood crashes after ruminating, take note. That's a sign. If you train your brain to recognize the sign, to be aware that this is something you don't enjoy, it will help you do less of it in the future.

- *Will this really matter a month or a year from now?* If you were looking back at this precise moment from the far-off future, would the conversation you're replaying in your head seem important enough to warrant the time and energy that are being sucked out of your day? You might borrow words of wisdom from Cher, who once said in an interview with *The New York Times* that the best advice she'd ever received was this: "If it doesn't matter in five years, it doesn't matter."

A week later, after trying these self-check-in techniques, Paola reaches out. Her favorite questions to ask herself when she's spiraling down into rumination are *Are my mental stories familiar?* and *Have I heard these same refrains many times before in my head?* "This moment of self-inquiry stops me cold," she tells me. "When my mind drama gets going, I realize it's the same refrains every time."

"What do the refrains sound like?" I ask.

"Why does Will say these things to me? Is he fundamentally broken? Will he ever grow up? Why didn't I see this coming when we got married? And did I really not want to have kids, or did I give that up because I wanted to get married? And what's wrong with him that he can't be compassionate when I'm vulnerable? Is he so selfish that he can't deal with the idea that one day he might not have his young, active, sexy partner in adventure?" She stops for a beat, pink breaking across her cheeks. "Conversely, what's wrong with me that I'm putting up with this, that I'm not speaking up? Why can't I find the right words to help him understand how I feel and what I really need from him?"

"Does practicing the checklist help stop that mind chatter?" I ask.

"It helps me to realize that even though my life is fine on the surface, underneath, I'm not fine. So examining my rumination is actually telling me something I need to know." She lets out a long burst of air from between her lips, as though just saying it is something of a relief.

Paola finds one other question in the checklist really helpful: *Am I searching for a solution where there is none?* Usually, that's exactly what she's doing, she fears. "I love Will. I love him a lot. I don't want to live my life without him. At this stage of life, I'm not about to run off and try to find some other life partner. So why do I spend so much time lost in my head about this?"

Paola has put her finger on the futility of the kind of ruminating she's been doing, and the way it can be a form of self-sabotage, which is preventing her from doing something useful about the situation she's in. Because the default mode network, when it goes into overdrive, is so good at keeping us running around in mental circles, versus offering insight and solutions, I'm going to call it your Inner Defeatist. When you ruminate, your Inner Defeatist is always fighting for your attention. *Tell me more about how they hurt me. Tell me more about what they think about me. Tell me more about what I did wrong, what they did wrong.* "This is how my rumination always seduces me and lures me in," Paola tells me. "It's almost like I *want* to feed my anger, as if that will somehow feel satisfying, even though it only makes me feel worse." Paola is right—the default mode network is best at tipping you into interior monologues that make you feel misunderstood, diminished, angry, unlovable, and wrapped in self-loathing.

And yet, once you've learned how to disrupt the default mode network's neural patterning you can begin to switch brain modes and enter a far healthier state—what researchers call *neural integration.* This is when all the parts of your brain start to hum together in a synchronized way so that your whole, clearheaded, insightful, ingenious mind machine works for you instead of against you. The more quickly and often you pull your brain's default mode out of lockdown, the more likely you'll be able to engage in what scientists call *neurorepair*—rewiring your neural circuitry.

This is important work. In the late nineteenth century, American philosopher William James wrote in his seminal book *The Principles of Psychology* that "we are spinning our own fates" and shaping our lives through our daily habits. As psychoanalyst Allen Wheelis puts it in his book *How People Change,* who we are is defined by our repetitive behaviors: "We are what we do." Though he says that for as "long as one lives, change is possible," he also acknowledges the difficulty of changing those behaviors: "Action which has been repeated over and over . . . tends to maintain itself, to resist change" and "the longer such behavior is continued the more force and authority it acquires."

So it's not so surprising that, even with her checklist, Paola admits that the gravitational pull of the old storylines is often too strong to resist. "The checklist helps, but it's not enough. Even though I know it's bad for my mood, my brain, I get sucked in every time."

Paola is, as I am, hungry for a deeper understanding of her ruminative tendencies. It's not enough to just shut off the spigot of rumination, which is difficult. She wants to know what her ruminations are trying to tell her beneath their churn and noise. "Why are all my pervasive thought loops about the same types of interactions, the same people and fears?" Paola wants strategies to help her not only stop ruminating but start processing her emotions in healthier, more constructive ways, so she can be proactive and find a better road forward—hopefully a road with Will walking alongside her—as they get older. "Otherwise, it's like playing Whac-A-Mole—I see I'm ruminating, but I have nowhere better for my brain to go."

I tell her I'm investigating this aspect of mind drama, too. And I've learned, after much research and self-experimentation, that certain strategies, when done in a step-by-step, neuroscience-based order, are remarkably, breathtakingly helpful. Indeed, it is only by truly listening to what our ruminations are trying to tell us about our stories, our self-beliefs and how we first came to form them, that we can experience life in its purer, more alive form. And who doesn't want to be lifted out of themselves into a greater sense of aliveness?

FIVE

What Messages Are Your Ruminations Sending You?

Cracking Your Personal Rumination Code

MY FRIEND ADA has worked in the film industry for over a decade as a set designer. Even though she's doing well in her work and has a lovely family, she's found herself, to use her word, languishing of late. Much of the problem, she realizes, is how exhausted she feels because of what's happening inside her head. Like Paola—and like so many of us—she finds herself replaying conflicts with her partner, whose habit of micro-managing her is increasingly causing tension between them. "I'll be in the kitchen chopping celery and my husband will come in and tell me I'm using the wrong knife, or the pieces of celery are too big for the stew, or that I've bought celery that isn't fresh enough. I'll say, 'Why are you being so critical?' And Carl will say, 'Why are you so defensive? I thought you'd want to know!'" And suddenly they're trading snipes, in an escalating battle Ada likens to "a duel with butter knives; they don't really cut, but they can hurt."

But the more pressing issue for Ada is that her daughter, Allie, is in the early throes of adolescence and is pulling away from her. When Ada, who is in her late thirties, was an adolescent, her mother "was so controlling and up in my stuff—she'd never heard the word *boundary*. Once I left for college at seventeen, I never came back. I couldn't bear to. The only way to win my mother's approval was to let her dictate everything and do whatever she told me to do—how to dress, how to wear my hair, who to be friends with." Ada set out to do things differently with her own daughter, encouraging her autonomy—only to now feel rejected by her.

Ada and I are chatting at a local wine bar after work. She is petite, her skin pale, her black hair cut short and sharp against her face. She wears a sleeveless black dress that fits her as if it were made just for her—and maybe it was. Ada is gifted with her sewing machine. There is something in the way she holds herself that always reminds me of old movies. A timeless grace smoothing over a kinetic nervous energy. Audrey Hepburn, maybe, though Ada would definitely laugh if I said so.

Recently, Ada has taken on more jobs and more clients. "I'm working seven days a week to save for college for Allie. It's coming up on us so fast! But no one seems to have any appreciation for how hard I'm pushing myself." Ada's husband, who is eleven years older, is semiretired and isn't making much money these days.

I ask Ada to take me inside of her ruminations around these familial dynamics, and she agrees. (Warning: It's not pretty, but it is very human.)

"I'll walk in the door after having been out of town for work, and Allie and Carl will be chatting about her debate team practice or something that happened with her friends, and Allie will clam up as I walk in, as if I'm getting in the way of their private conversation. If I ask her questions, she says, 'Everything is *fine*, Mom!' I feel so diminished and rejected. And suddenly, I'm stewing as I unpack my bags; I can't stop replaying it. It's childish, I know. I know I'm the parent! But this old tape gets going. . . . *Here I am working so hard to take care of everyone, provide for everyone, please everyone, and no one cares about me or what I need."*

These thoughts "feel like striking a match; they rekindle memories of incidents in my childhood when my mother was so intrusive that I wanted nothing more than to get away from her. Does Allie feel like that about me? And then I feel guilty for resenting her for wanting space. Am I just like my mom, even though that's the last person I want to be?" Often, Ada moves from her resentment of her mother's intrusiveness to her resentment of Carl's micromanaging, and she starts to smolder, her thoughts tumbling out in the way they do when people have been sitting with them for too long. Every so often, she reaches up and pushes her hair back from her forehead as she speaks, her hands moving almost absently. "Who does he think he is telling me how to cook? I've been cooking dinner for all of us for fifteen years, and until he started to make dinner when I'm out of town on business, he never had any complaints. Suddenly, he criticizes everything I do the minute I step in the kitchen. And why am I such a doormat that I can't stand up for myself and tell him to stop it?"

Then the wheel of rumination spins back to her daughter: "Allie used to tell me everything. During her first twelve years, I put my career on hold to stay home with her. But now that I've gone back to work full-time—so that we can pay for her college—it's like she's trying to punish me for being gone. I'm trying to give her space, but she just keeps distancing herself from me, and that makes me try to force my way back into her world. It's so painful, because it means despite my efforts not to let this mother-daughter pattern repeat, it is repeating, and this time on *my* watch."

This gets Ada thinking about her relationship with her mother again and how resentful she had been of her mother's attempt to control her: "Growing up, if I wanted my mother's nod of affection, I had to turn myself into a pretzel and be the kind of daughter she envisioned. It's the same message I'm getting from Allie: I'm not lovable for who I really am, and I guess I never will be."

And round and round and round Ada's merry-go-round of rumination goes.

Though everyone's circumstances are different, these kinds of feelings, which have at their heart our existential longing to know, in some tender, essential part of ourselves, that we matter to those around us, are what set so many people to ruminating. This is why so many of the portraits of my interviewees' ruminations sound similar. What sparks their ruminations varies, and what they need to do about them also varies, but the underlying feeling is often the same.

Recently, as Ada's work hours have increased and with them the amount of stress she is feeling, the movies swirling in her head have become more overwhelming. "I feel sad that I spend so much time replaying difficult moments with people I love. My daughter won't be living at home that much longer. My mother isn't going to live forever. My husband is a good man, but he's driving me crazy. My life, and our time together, is speeding by. And what am I doing? Listening to stories in my head. It's like there's this little monster in my head who, when she feels injured, roars and stomps around, lost in her ungenerous thoughts about everybody, including myself. The other day, it hit me how much of my time that little monster devours, and I just started sobbing."

Ada knows I've been working on a project in which I'm investigating the science and strategies that might help her tame her "little monster."

"Once you learn how to put a pause on the movies running in your rumination," I offer, "you can slow down the action long enough to examine their storylines and find out what they are trying to tell you. I've got some techniques that can help you to do that, I think."

What if, I pose to Ada, our struggles—our ruminations—stem from parts of ourselves carrying pain and parts protecting that pain? And what if we can decode what that pain is whispering to us in ways that help us understand our wounds and the thought patterns they give rise to? What if our stickiest ruminations are encoded with information that can help us finally heal those wounds?

"*How?*" Ada asks, an edge of desperation in her voice.

The MIST Technique

One of the most powerful approaches I've found—one that works remarkably quickly and has saved me time and again—is a technique I call *MIST*, an acronym I'll unpack below. I developed this framework after twenty-five years of working with neuroscientists and psychologists, based on our evolving understanding of how the default mode network gives rise to our stickiest ruminations, as well as an understanding of what is necessary to make shifts happen in that network.

To validate this science-based approach, I reach out to Ruth Lanius. I want to be sure my framework for MIST aligns with how the default mode network engenders our ruminations, as well as how we can begin to unlatch ourselves from its machinations. When I share MIST with her, Lanius sees and corroborates its value as a gentle tool for self-inquiry and self-awareness. "This is how the default mode network serves up our stories to us," she tells me. "And it beautifully connects what I do in the lab with what patients are feeling and experiencing in their lives."

In my workshops, I've seen time and time again how the practice of MIST helps individuals to shift out of a ruminative state into a proactive and helpful state—and in a surprisingly short time. I've learned that real change begins not with forceful willpower but with gentle awareness of our mental patterns. It's a process rooted in both curiosity and humility. (That said, it bears repeating that if you are struggling with pressing mental health concerns, please share those with a trusted health practitioner.)

◆ ◆ ◆ ◆

Before I show you how the MIST Technique can help you to reverse engineer your ruminations for deep and even profound self-reflection, it will help to have a deeper understanding of precisely how your default mode network works. As I mentioned in chapter 1, the default mode network is composed of three different brain areas—the *posterior cingulate cortex*, which, with the help of your brain's memory center, the hippocampus, recalls memories and images from across your life and interprets them in ways that, over time, shape your story of who you believe yourself to be; the *dorsal medial prefrontal cortex*, which helps you regulate difficult feelings and emotions, put things in perspective, and self-regulate; and the *parietal lobe*, which generates somatic and physical sensations in your body.

These three areas communicate with you through three different modalities—your mental imagery, intense emotions, and bodily sensations. Your *mental imagery*, often in the form of a movie reel you have seen many times before (whether it's of something that happened a lifetime or an hour ago), can deliver you into hurtful memories from your past and project alarming scenarios about who and what might harm you in the future. The *intense emotions* you feel amplify the power of these mental movies, much as the musical score in a film does. And your *somatic bodily sensations*, which can be anything, including shortness of breath, a stabbing pain in the gut, heart palpitations, or muscles tightening, are churned up by the anxiety created by these stressful mental images and emotions.

For each of us, the imagery, emotions, and bodily sensations that characterize our ruminations are distinct and constitute what I call your *personal rumination code*. The way to crack this code, to escape your ruminative state, is by describing these familiar images, feelings, and sensations in words. Labeling each of them with shorthand names you will instantly recognize can become your portal to escape, helping you to make a remarkably quick exit.

Finding the words for all of this is part of the work, and

because doing that requires some serious self-examination, it may seem hard at first. The poet Rumi once wrote, "Do you pay regular visits to yourself?" For most of us, the answer is—not often enough. Research shows that although 95 percent of us think we're self-aware, only about 10 to 15 percent of us are. We're so bogged down in our stories about ourselves that we can't see behind the scrim of our mind drama. We get mired in the intimate melodrama of our ruminations, but we don't know how to step back and distance ourselves from them to see them for what they are. And yet, when properly heard, our ruminations are an invitation to tend to the fearful, anxious, exiled, grieving, angry, unheard parts of ourselves. That is the work we are setting out to do here.

Using the steps of MIST will help you to recognize and name your difficult feelings and to accept them, while not giving them power over how you spend the remaining precious moments of your life. In the end, rumination is often about resistance. Although it feels like an immersion into our suffering, it's actually a means of avoidance, a way of suppressing our subconscious emotions, which only makes our mind drama stronger. This recalls writer Bertrand Russell's words: "Every kind of fear grows worse by not being looked at. The effort of turning away one's thoughts becomes a tribute to the horribleness of the specter from which one is averting one's gaze." By asking us to name our feelings, MIST puts us gently, reverently, in touch with the emotions we are avoiding, so we can begin to process them at last.

In short, you can use MIST as a powerful tool to defeat your Inner Defeatist. Your default mode network replays your ruminative thoughts and corrosive self-beliefs because your pain hasn't been acknowledged and processed. When you recognize, honor, and name your rumination pattern with granular language—in a way that speaks to the role each area of the default mode network plays in perpetuating your mind drama—you free both yourself and your mind from spinning on repeat. This simple act, as we'll see in part 3, allows your brain to open up, on a neurobiological level, to wiser thinking so you can choose more productive and joyful ways to spend your priceless mental energy.

Practicing MIST

The MIST acronym consists of

M for ***Mental movies***—the imagery and montages you see in your mind

I for ***Intense inner emotions***—the feelings evoked by the mental movies

S for the ***Sensations you experience in your body***—the sensations that arise in response to the mental movies and the accompanying emotions

T for ***Tie it all together***—to gain empowering self-insights that might otherwise remain opaque and hidden from your view

Here is the four-step process of MIST.

1. M. Recognize your familiar parade of mental movies. Many of the mental images and stories you ruminate about are repeats. You've probably thought about them many times before—which is why some researchers call them *thought worms.*

A destructive core belief is often the main theme of these mental movies and montages: *I did something wrong. Something's wrong with me. I always mess up. I'm not capable or good enough.*

But when you give these brain movies a name—"Here is my story of why no one ever helps me" or "Here is my story of how I'm always left out" or "Here is my story of how people dismiss me"—you hit Pause on your film reel and begin to extricate yourself from the grasp of your Inner Defeatist. (One note here: For some people, detailed memories or images might not arise; you might simply experience flashes of something sensed or felt—the vibration of something old and familiar—while specific details remain obscure. That's okay, too.)

*2. I. **Name your intense inner emotions.*** Left unnamed, the intense emotions you feel, which generally sync up with your mental imagery, can be quite painful. Naming them, however, deflates their intensity. This idea of naming emotions to lessen their impact—"Name it to tame it"—was first developed by Dan Siegel, MD, in response to studies using fMRI scans, which showed that when we accurately name and identify emotions with very precise words (versus in broad, general terms) our brains shift in ways that help us to self-regulate.

As effective as this is, when you string together the names that apply to your emotions, with the name you gave to your mental movie, the strategy becomes even more powerful.

For purposes of the MIST Technique, the names you give the emotions that correlate to your mental movie are very much up to you and what feels true to you. They can be as silly or serious as you want. So come up with language that will help you recognize them instantly: "Here is my old familiar fear ball." Or "Here is my cloud of dread." Or "Here's my tsunami of resentment." Or "Here's the lake of misery I keep drowning in."

Once you've done that, and you put it together with your movie name, it will sound something like this: "Here is my old story of how I'm always left out, which leaves me drowning in my lake of misery."

You may be skeptical about the point of doing this, but it's actually very powerful, because it lets you see the connection between your feelings and your mental imagery. The default mode network registers this shift in perspective, too. You're putting your thoughts in a new arrangement. Making this connection becomes another weapon in your arsenal against the Inner Defeatist.

*3. S. **Observe the sensations in your body.*** Note the raw, physical sensations you feel in your body in conjunction with your mental movies and your emotions. Many of the feelings our ruminations churn up—fear, anxiety, anger, and more—become somatic experiences, meaning they are felt in the body, not just the mind. And just as the emotions can be hard to escape, the accompanying physical sensations can overwhelm us, too (as they did me when I became so upset about the British researcher who was planning to use my work in his own publication).

Simply put, if we think distressing thoughts long enough, our bodies become anxious, too. But it's also the case that our physical sensations can become palpable before we ever register whatever emotions we are feeling and can influence our mental state.

As Ruth Lanius explains, "Visceral sensations, including body temperature, thirst, nausea, abdominal sensations, all inform your positive and negative emotions. Your inner bodily sensations converge at the base of your brain, in the brain stem, which initiates initial reactions to your environment before you're even aware it's happening. These somatic sensations can also reach the higher emotional centers of your brain," where they can be accessed at a conscious level. When we "consciously appraise these raw, visceral sensations and identify them, we can act with intention to process them."

The process of discerning exactly where your difficult feelings are manifesting in your body is known as *interoception*, and it is crucial to helping you escape your cyclical, brooding thoughts. The sensations you feel may have been catalyzed by something that is upsetting you—the ominous discussion you had with your boss at your annual review, the argument you had on the phone with a friend, some worrisome news you received from your doctor—but if you can locate them and find language to describe them—"Here's that shoulder and jaw tension," or "Here's that belly-churning feeling again," or "Here's that ache in my solar plexus"—you can metabolize them and help yourself escape them.

4. T. Tie it all together. Now you're really getting somewhere. By tying together the three different types of awareness that correspond to the three areas of the default mode network and the distinct experiences they give rise to, you can arrive at a self-understanding that may be profound.

"Here's my old story of how I'm always left out, which drowns me in misery and makes my chest ache" is an insight you can build on. Just the simple act of naming can enable you to intercept and stop your rumination feedback loop cold, unlocking the hold it has on your nervous system.* Now you have a little space and distance from your thoughts. You're standing six feet back, observing rather than inhabiting the mind drama that has so regularly derailed you. This offers you a golden moment of perspective. And that small moment of perspective is a game changer.

From here, another awareness arises: You never signed up for this warped, distorted view of yourself. It's not who you are. It's a product of messages that were very likely inculcated in you at such an early age you didn't have any choice about accepting them. But you do have a choice now. These old destructive self-beliefs and the corrosive ruminations they engender are not yours to carry anymore.

MIST in Action

Shortly after my conversation with Ada, I sent her the MIST Technique. When I next touched base with her, I asked her how it went.

"When I'm ruminating, I see the same mental slideshows in my head, scenes of my husband criticizing me, or my mother inserting herself and her opinions into my life, or my daughter shutting me out. It's a theme. An old movie playing

* One note: For individuals who have experienced extremely severe trauma (which might include individuals with PTSD and CPTSD), the default mode network can behave differently. For more on this, see chapter 12.

the same clips I've watched a thousand times. They bring up the same intense emotions—fear that if I say something about how other people's words or actions make me feel, they'll tell me I'm imagining it, or I'm the one who's to blame, or turn on me in some passive-aggressive way. Carl will tell me I'm attacking him and stomp out of the kitchen. My mom will tell me I've hurt her feelings, and suddenly, I'll be the ungrateful daughter. Allie will roll her eyes and go to her room and slam the door and shut me out even more. And that dredges up this old feeling that I'm not a good mom; not the mom Allie wants me to be. Even when I give all of me, I'm not enough as I am. If I'm not what my mother or my daughter wanted, I must be fundamentally flawed, dislikable. And if I want to keep relationships with these people intact, I must stay very, very small and minimize my true feelings, while focusing my energy on taking care of them and what they need, instead of figuring out what I need. When I ask myself, *Where do I feel this in my body?* I feel my heart hurtling out of my chest. I hear my pulse pounding in my ears, my head." Ada pauses to pull out a piece of notepaper on which she's written down the personal rumination code this has led her to. "When I tie it together, I get, *Here is my old story about how I'm unlikable and have to stay small and ignore my true feelings unless I want to be alone, which makes my heart bang in my head.*"

Once Ada stepped back and let her rumination reveal itself with words, images, and insights, she "had had that click of awareness when everything snaps into place. I realized these are the same feelings I've struggled to process forever." Ada saw, just as urgently, how her silence wasn't serving her. "I don't want to live my life afraid to say what I'm feeling out of fear they'll stop loving me."

Ada is continuing to use the MIST Technique to good avail. "It's not an intellectual experience. It's an experiential, a feeling state." In her explorations, she's been able to go deeper into the bodily sensations that arise at challenging moments, making more nuanced connections between those sensations and her emotions. When she's replaying difficult conversations with her daughter, "I feel a band tighten around my upper abdomen, like a vise, kind of where I'd put my hand on my belly when I was pregnant." When her husband micromanages or critiques her, "panic spreads from my heart into my upper chest, into my head." And when she gets lost in thought spirals about the resentment she still feels toward her mother, "a crushing weight falls across my shoulders and upper back, like I'm carrying a load too heavy to bear."

This discernment, she tells me, has not only increased her dexterity at sidestepping her mind drama in real time, but it's made her "want to evolve. I've been putting the expectation on the people around me to notice my unfilled needs and fill them; to resolve things in me only I can resolve. When they don't, I resent them." This makes Ada wonder, more broadly, what she is role modeling for Allie. "How can I model for Allie how to express herself as a woman in this world if I'm not speaking up for myself?"

Ada's work with the MIST Technique has led her to change the way she responds to Carl when he is mansplaining in the kitchen. "I tell him, very calmly, 'I'm not looking for any advice right now. I've got this.' Or I ask him, 'Are you volunteering to chop the carrots?' He might balk and say, 'I thought you'd want to know!' But even if I'm met with a poor response, speaking up feels better than letting him get under my skin." The beauty of speaking up, Ada tells me, is that "there is no residual drama inside my head. When I say what I think, I don't ruminate afterward, because I haven't betrayed myself by staying silent in the first place. That's been a real eye-opener."

What a change this has made in her—and her relationships—was revealed early one Saturday morning when Ada was about to drive Allie to a debate tournament an hour away. Carl asked which route Ada planned to take, and every time Ada started to explain how she planned to get there, he interrupted to say, "No, no, I don't think so." The third time, Ada turned around and said, "Thanks, but I've researched this, and I've got it." Carl's jaw dropped before he caught himself and said, "Okay."

A few minutes later, when Ada was alone with Allie in the car, Allie told her, "Mom, good for you for standing up to Dad! That was great!" She vented to Ada, then, about how irritating it was to be around boys and men who "shut women down." Allie told her, "I'm not going to marry anyone who does that shit!" Ada wondered if perhaps on some level, "Allie has been waiting for *me* to grow up? Have I been so caught up all these years in my self-judgy, wounded, put-upon-woman thought spirals that I haven't been someone she felt she could turn to? Isn't this another version of what my mother did to me? Made me fear *her* moods so much that I just withdrew? Maybe Allie has been waiting for me to show her I know how to take care of myself, so she knows it's safe to voice her feelings to me; that I can handle her emotions. I could be wrong, but if I'm right, it's quite a revelation."

Paola also gave MIST a try one day when she was feeling utterly frustrated with Will because he was rushing her to get ready to leave for an event much earlier than necessary, as he so often did, and calling her Slowpoke, a nickname he often uses in such situations. "When I thought about my mental imagery, I realized other memories were getting churned up—not just about Will but from much earlier in my life. Growing up, I had five siblings. My parents were good parents, but we were pretty much left on our own. I was the youngest and got the brunt of the teasing, some of it good-natured, but a lot of it was incredibly hurtful. Or maybe it was just the constancy of it, never feeling I could relax because someone would say or do something mean."

Paola tells me that after she read *Charlotte's Web* in grade school and refused to eat bacon, her siblings teased her mercilessly and started calling her "the runt." They'd routinely do things like swoop in and take her piece of cake off her plate, then stare at her and dare her to say anything. It was as constant as it was tiring. "My parents didn't know, and I didn't tell, because tattling would have made it worse. It was just normal life in my house as the 'runt.'" One day, all five siblings went speeding off on their bikes, and Paola desperately tried to keep up. At first, the sister closest to her in age stayed beside her, but then she, too, sped up, leaving Paola behind. Paola lagged so far behind that no one was there to see when the front wheel of her bike caught in a pothole, and she went flying over the handlebars. "It took them a long time to notice that I wasn't with them and come back and find me on the side of the road."

As she paid close attention to this mental imagery, Paola noticed intense emotions bubbling up. "I started crying and I asked myself, *Why am I crying? I never cry!* All these feelings I'd never expressed before came right to the surface. That feeling that no one looks out for me. No one cares about me. I can't count on anyone. I didn't grow up in a way that allowed me to express feelings like that. If I'd been emotional or vulnerable, I wouldn't have heard the end of it from my siblings."

As for her bodily sensations, Paola felt her silencing as a pain across her shoulders. She noticed that when she was ruminating, she hunched forward, her chest caved in, head tucked down, as if to protect herself. Finally, when she tied her mental movies, intense emotions, and somatic sensations together, Paola came up with this: "*Here's my old story of how people disappear on me or diminish me, which makes me feel abandoned and grief-stricken, like I have to hunker down to protect myself, and freeze.*"

"For the first time," Paola tells me, "I realized I hadn't been feeling my feelings. I'd been ruminating about who said or did what instead of listening to what was really going on with me." She became aware that ruminating isn't an immersion in feeling; instead, it's a way of suppressing her feelings about what she needs. But once she brought her attention to where her feelings were lodged in her body, Paola realized the mental images, intense emotions, and somatic sensations that comprise her ruminations had something crucial to tell her. "I understood why I was feeling conflicted about my marriage. When Will is rushing me or making fun of me or ignoring the fact that I'm in pain and could use a bit of empathy, I feel like that girl on the bike—expected to keep up, and if I don't, too bad for me, he might just whiz off and leave me on the side of the road when I get older. I don't trust Will to be mature enough for me to be vulnerable with him."

When Paola allowed these feelings to arise and emerge, some of their power dissolved. "All those emotions were energy I was suppressing. That energy was getting twisted inside me, obscuring me from clarity. Now I have a better sense of my whole story, and tapping into that makes me feel compassion for myself—the girl I was, and the woman I am now, trying to figure all this out before I'm ninety."

Georgia O'Keeffe once wrote, "Making your unknown known is the important thing." The MIST Technique works, I think, because it does that. When we do this work, we weave new threads between our stories and the pain we carry, and we make our patterns transparent to ourselves. We're able to catch ourselves before we jump into our old ruts of thinking, to make the kind of external observations about ourselves that a kind friend or therapist might make, and use that awareness to begin to change our patterns. As Steve Jobs said, "Creativity is just connecting things." When you make connections by using MIST, you are actually doing something that is genuinely creative.

It isn't always easy, however. It takes practice. It takes a willingness to look at your pain. But either way—whether you decode your ruminations or not—your pain is going to come up. Physician and trauma expert Gabor Maté, MD, often says that your pain will arise whether you suppress your feelings or feel and voice them. Both are painful, yes, but only the latter will set you free. Or, to put it in Brené Brown's words, "We can choose courage, or we can choose comfort, but we can't have both. Not at the same time."

SIX

Your Understory

What Role Is It Playing in Your Life Today?

WHEN YOU LEARN to decode your stickiest recurring thoughts, you're investigating the understory beneath the surface story of your life. Sometimes it's relatively easy to trace the roots of the stories clamoring inside our heads, but not always. It can be a lot harder than it sounds. In one 2017 study of students, 90 percent "reported not having had any previous knowledge of the links between thoughts, feelings, and behavior." We rarely learn this growing up—instead, we internalize the negative stories we have learned to tell ourselves and come to believe they are true, without questioning them.

Amanda Ripley, a cofounder of the group Good Conflict, an organization that offers workshops to help people develop the habits and skills of good conflict, employs a useful technique to teach people how challenging past experiences can ignite powerful feelings in the present—an important step toward having said "good conflict." Ripley says if you're unsure how your painful mental stories link to your origin story of "not belonging," simply ask yourself, "When was the first time I remember feeling like I didn't belong?" Or "When was the first time I experienced fear of conflict?"

Maybe it was when a parent was in an ill temper and lashed out at you for no reason, and you felt afraid because the parent who had attacked you was also the person you most relied on to protect you. Maybe you watched your parents fling verbal zingers at each other and developed a sense of hypervigilance, as if by continually surveilling the situation for signs of a coming altercation, you could keep them together. Maybe you were teased and tormented by your siblings and peeked out your bedroom door to make sure none of them were around before you went down to the kitchen on Sunday mornings, or you were bullied by kids in the neighborhood and started walking home from school a different way to avoid them.

I suggested to Sam, the young med student, that he ask himself this question—*When was the first time I felt fear about conflict?*—to help him better understand his ruminations around his med school mentor. He came away with a profound revelation: His mental movies might start with resentments toward his adviser, but they always brought back split-second memories of scenes with his bipolar and sometimes volatile father. "I think my first experiences of conflict occurred when I was really little. Once, after I left my bike in the rain, he gave it to a neighbor's son. Another time, I was five or six, and I forget what I did, but he went storming outside and kicked down the snowman we'd made. Another time, he took a toy truck I'd been playing with and dropped it in the toilet and said, 'Do you still want it?'" Sam's father never apologized. Instead, he used to mock Sam for getting upset, telling Sam's mom, "He's too sensitive. He's a mama's boy. I need to toughen him up."

"My mom always kept me safe, and out of the way, whenever he was manic. Twice, things got so bad we left and lived with her parents. But she always tried to minimize my fear, telling me, 'You know your dad loves you, and this will pass. He's only hurting himself.' But that felt so invalidating. It also didn't feel true."

Eventually, Sam tells me, his father got the help he needed, and he now has the skills to regulate his emotions. "But those first ten or twelve years of my life were all about conflict—my dad's rage, his fits, my mother telling him if he didn't get help, we'd leave. . . . I didn't ever feel safe when my father was in the house. The minute I heard the front door open at the end of the day, I felt afraid. I froze."

When Sam finds himself ruminating about how critical his adviser is of him, if he practices the MIST Technique, he's able to observe from a distance what comes into his mind and body, and also to see how his ruminations about the present keep spitting up mental movies of his father's fits of rage. Watching the intense emotions that course through his mind as he replays those scenes, Sam can identify the destructive messages being sent to him, then and now, about how he is supposed to respond—and in how he's been programmed to react. "I have to agree with and believe what I'm being told, even if I know it's not true or right, or something bad will happen." And that leads to a rage that he hasn't—until now—realized he was feeling. As for his somatic sensations, Sam feels them as a "tension and pain through my jawline and my eyes, as if I were clenching my teeth and squeezing my eyes shut."

When Sam ties it all together, he gets: "*Here is my old fear of how people who hold power over me can torment me whenever they want, which makes me feel angry and afraid and resentful, and then my whole face clenches.*"

Recognizing how his understory gets reactivated in his default mode network by his professor has helped Sam see that he's given up his power to his professor and allowed him to make Sam feel guilty about his uncertainty about what he wants to specialize in. He had no choices when he was a child with a rageful, unpredictable father. But thanks to the connections he's been able to make through MIST, which have opened his eyes to alternate ways of interpreting and responding to events, he knows he does have choices now. So he's decided that he will take whatever time he needs to choose his specialty, without feeling pressured by his mentor.

If You Feel Stuck or Need Help to Access Your Understory

When Virginia and I next touch base, she, too, is intrigued by trying to connect her origin story with her ruminations. But she was finding it difficult to use the MIST Technique, so I shared with her an exercise I use when teaching workshops. A gentle way to dive into better understanding your origin story is to draw a rough floor plan of the home you lived in when you were a child. You may be surprised by what comes up when you do this very simple exercise.

If you want to explore this for yourself, grab a piece of paper and a pencil and begin to sketch (these are just rough sketches, no artistic skills required!). Here are some guidelines that might be helpful:

1. If you moved around a lot or lived in more than one house, draw the floor plan of the home that brings up the most memories for you.
2. Add three to six details, or more, if you like, such as the kitchen table where you had dinner with your family, the closet where you kept your toys, the front of the refrigerator, whatever comes to mind. The more details, the better. Do you remember the color of your closet door? How many chairs were at the table? What photos or magnets were on the front of the refrigerator?
3. Now sketch the exterior of the house, showing the front or back door, the yard, street, or sidewalk outside, and a few details about what was there—a swing set, a tree you could see from your bedroom window, a chain-link fence, the shop across the street where your parents sent you on errands or where you bought your comic books—whatever you best remember about your surroundings.

   A mix of feelings and memories may emerge from these details. Some memories may be happy and evoke a sense of safety; others may fill you with a sense of loss, sadness, even fear. Just let the feelings surface and know that whatever you are feeling is perfectly normal.

The first time I sketched the floor plan of my own childhood home, I drew my father's blue easy chair. I have a lot of happy memories of watching TV with my dad as he sat there. I also drew the bookshelves and stereo system in our living room. After my father died, I often sat in the living room listening to the Broadway musicals we'd listened to together, and reading the books we'd read together, missing him terribly.

4. Now, take a moment to reflect on and write about the feelings that came up for you as you drew your childhood home. What did daily life feel like for you growing up there? Jot down whatever feelings and emotions arise for you.
5. Pay attention to any new awareness that arises about how your childhood might still be affecting you now, and commit to working on better understanding this connection so that you can further your own healing.

When Virginia experimented with this, she had a profound experience. One of the things she drew in her floor plan was her father's painting studio. Her father was a very successful painter, and beginning in high school, she often went to his studio to show him her own artistic endeavors, which her teachers told her showed real talent. But whenever he deigned to look up from his work to look at hers, he would be "entirely dismissive," telling her she was no artist and she should focus her energies elsewhere. She also sketched the table in the dining room of her childhood home, the setting for a memorable scene in which her father critiqued her, which took place when she was visiting her parents for the Christmas holidays. As they sat down to eat, her father told her, "One day, maybe you'll be a beautiful woman and can find a husband." She was thirty at the time, and this became a refrain he repeated many times until she did get married some years later.

It was only when she drew the floor plan that these memories surfaced, helping her to connect her present-day ruminations about various people who she feels have belittled her with her sense of being, as she put it to me, "both unseen in childhood and a failure in adulthood." She understands that her ruminations are a reversion to that time, and "to that deepest core belief that I am not lovable, I don't matter and never will."

"Does this realization help you?" I ask.

Virginia says something then that I find very moving. "I think I always assumed that once I'd succeeded in my work and raised a family, I would be able to turn my hand to painting again, which I've wanted to do ever since college. And I am doing that. But instead of enjoying it, I'm letting criticism in the workshop get to me, so I just keep ruminating about whether I'm any good. Doing the floor plan took me back to my father's studio and suddenly gave me new information about why I'm being so hard on myself, and also why it's so hard for me to hear any criticism. Painful as it was, it was a very freeing realization. I don't have to keep visiting that studio to be told I have no talent. It gives me real hope that I can let go of those old judgments."

Honoring the Signal Fires from Your Past

As was true for Virginia, our understory is often as familial as it is familiar. Our rumination is a signal fire from our past, asking us to notice the reasons behind our overwhelming feelings, so we can touch compassionately into that vulnerable, wounded part of ourselves that is still experiencing these emotions. When Paola talks about the pain of being left behind by her siblings when she went flying over the handles of her bike and seeing how that relates to her fear that her husband, Will, won't be the partner she needs as they age, she is touching into the familiar—and familial—understory that fuels her ruminations. When Ada talks about how her daughter is pulling away, and how that makes her feel she's not good enough to be loved by even her own child, and how that echoes feeling she was not worthy enough to be loved by her own mother, she is unveiling the familial understory that gives rise to her Inner Defeatist, spewing its familiar self-beliefs. Virginia, Ada, Paola, and Sam have all learned to connect their understory with their overstory, and feel more whole. For Virginia, this practice is like "gently removing the age and smoke damage from the surface of an oil painting; if you do it carefully, you can reveal what's really underneath."

Virginia (as I have) has found (as I have) that when she's particularly swept up in her ruminations, she often has to repeat this process: "It's not a one-and-done." She'll start to crack her code only to "get sucked right back in again." (This, I remind her, is because it's the nature of the default mode network to keep delivering us back to the same stories where we dig among those ancient ruins for answers, even when none are to be found there.) This is especially true when Virginia has had recent interactions with less-than-supportive peers. I reassure her it's perfectly normal to have to repeat these steps and for it to take many rounds before we loosen the grip of our Inner Defeatist. We can restart this sequence as many times as we need to. Each time we do, we're retraining our default mode network to let go of our ruminations more quickly, and with less effort, in the future.

Over time, we're teaching our brains something else: When we feel highly activated, because something old in us has been ignited, we have options. It's important, when we feel stressed, that we feel some locus of control over external events. MIST is a way of developing *an internal locus of control*—the feeling that we have a sense of agency over our mental state—that we can draw on whenever we need to. We stop underestimating our ability to cope. We know we have the tools to prevent external events and interactions from destroying our equilibrium.

◆ ◆ ◆ ◆

Once you realize your Inner Defeatist regurgitates painful emotions from earlier life events because you were not able to fully process those emotions when they first occurred, you open the doorway to hope and change. New, empowering realizations might emerge. For Sam, practicing MIST allowed him to see "these old beliefs were placed in me when I was too young to sign on or agree to them. I didn't sign on for this!" Suddenly, your runaway thoughts not only make sense, but they now fall under your locus of control.

I have one last story I want to share with you about using MIST. Sometimes, the idea that what's happening now is connected to what happened long ago can feel far-fetched—especially when the pain and confusion you're experiencing seem completely disconnected from your past. This was true for a woman I'll call Devon, who approached me after a workshop I gave for parents of teens. She was consumed by the fallout from a thirty-five-year friendship that had imploded, affecting her entire family. "It's all I can think about—the things she and her daughter have said and done to hurt me and my daughter. But I also have these beautiful memories from when our kids were little. My brain ricochets between my grief and my rage." Devon understood the MIST Technique, but when she tried to use it to work through her mind drama about this situation, she couldn't find a link to her own past memories or experiences.

I invited her to share more.

Devon's story unfolded: She and her friend met in college, settled in the same city, and had their first children around the same time. Their daughters grew up together—same schools, sleepovers, even joint family vacations. In middle school, Devon's daughter was accepted to a magnet school; her friend's daughter wasn't. The next year, Devon, a learning specialist, helped her friend's daughter with her application. Once admitted, the dynamic shifted: "Even though my daughter brought her into her friend group, she started leaving my daughter out. First, she cut her out of group chats, then sleepovers. At school, she'd only talk to her when the 'cooler kids' weren't around." The classic sting of exclusion. Devon's daughter eventually found a new, supportive friend group. But in senior year, her former best friend spread a cruel rumor about her—something private she'd learned during their childhood sleepovers—turning it into gossip in group chats and on social media. The school intervened, threatening suspension for bullying, but Devon's friend pressured the school to let their daughter do community service instead.

"This isn't the first time they've excused her behavior," Devon said, her anger palpable. To make matters worse, both girls applied to their mothers' shared alma mater for college. Devon's friend "cashed in a chit"—her sister was on the admissions board. Devon's daughter, a top student, didn't get in. Devon was convinced her ex-friend had sabotaged her daughter's chances. "I can't get over it. My friends are furious, too; they've watched this dynamic unfold for years. It's practically all we talk about." Still, she added, "I'm not sure MIST can help me with this—my childhood was pretty solid; there was no 'big life adversity.' Couldn't all my feelings just be from the anger I feel at being betrayed after three decades of friendship?"

I told her, "That's a fair question." But I think part of the problem might lie in the fact that we so often misunderstand what the term *adversity* means. At its core, childhood adversity isn't just about what happened to you—it's also about how you felt. It's those moments when you had to stay vigilant, bracing yourself for unpredictable relationships or events. It's the experience of not feeling safe or seen, while also feeling you couldn't turn to a trusted adult who would comfort you and help you make sense of what was happening.

I asked, "Does that resonate with you?"

Devon flushed. She admitted that as a teen, she and her twin sister were often at odds. Her sister was more athletic, more popular. Devon excelled academically, but in high school, that didn't seem to matter. When their parents weren't around, her sister would call her *fat, dorky, unpopular*—listing all the reasons boys didn't like her—starting at her "big" feet and going all the way up to her "pimply face" and "limp brown hair." Her sister would also regularly lie to their parents about where she was, and Devon would be left to back up her lies. "She lorded her popularity over me. I felt I had to keep all her secrets. I guess I did feel hypervigilant around her—but mostly, I felt ill-used. We're close now—she's even apologized for being a 'brat.' But back then, it was like my best friend had turned on me."

"Does any of that feel familiar?" I asked. "Is there an echo, a vibration, of that old hurt in what you and your daughter have experienced?"

Devon shook her head in disbelief, as if seeing it for the first time. "So it's like, 'Here's my old story: *Someone I trust turns on me—or by proxy, on my daughter, which, honestly, is even more painful—which makes my jaw clench and makes me feel bitter and enraged*'?"

I really didn't need to say anything in return. But I did want Devon to know one more thing before she left—something that it will be helpful for you to know, too. When she recounted her story, I was struck by her comment that the fallout from this friendship was practically the only thing she and her friends talked about. On the one hand, studies show that when women talk through things with other women and receive support, care, and validation—what researchers call *tending and befriending*—it's enormously good for us. It sends a potent safety signal from our brains throughout our whole bodies. Our heart rates slow as levels of the feel-good, bonding hormone oxytocin rise, and stress hormones like cortisol drop. But there is a flip side. Replaying our injuries with friends, collecting more evidence of how we've been wronged, stacking up reasons to vilify someone, and rehashing it all ad nauseam—even when another's actions are reprehensible—can quickly become what's called *co-rumination.* And co-rumination is toxic for our bodies and minds. It keeps our pain alive, spinning our default mode network into ever-stickier, more persistent mind drama—making it much harder to escape.

Devon half laughed, half nodded. "I wish I'd known this a year ago!"

I can't promise that using MIST will apply to every situation in which you find yourself lost in mind drama. But usually, if we listen to what our mind drama has to tell us, we will hear the vibration of something old—that essential longing to belong, to matter, especially with the people whom we have loved and who we thought would always have our backs. Sometimes, the echoes of these old wounds are so subtle it's hard to recognize them—especially when the pain feels new and the past seems far away. But even when we can't immediately see the connection, those early experiences can quietly shape how we feel, react, and heal.

So where does this leave me, with my own story? Like all of us, I have multiple patterns of rumination, depending on the memory or event, the people involved in the story I tell myself about that event, and what my feelings, in reaction, may be excavating from the annals of my childhood.

When I crack the code of my ruminations and think about how my understory meets my overstory, and the ways that my core beliefs about myself were formed as a child, profound insights emerge. One mental pattern that MIST uncovered has to do with my role in my family after my father died. At the time, my mother was, as I have said, understandably overwhelmed by grief, by rage at the unfairness of having her young husband taken from her, and being left to raise four children alone, and by panic about whether she would be able to provide for us. The implicit contract everyone in the family agreed to—including me—was that, as the only girl, it was my responsibility to stay by my mother's side and tend to her distress. So I learned, almost overnight, to suppress my own feelings. Whenever I did attempt to express something I was worried about, or share an opinion, my mother's most common response was to say, in an exhausted voice, "No one wants to hear what you have to say." She was so perpetually drained that even the sound of my voice seemed to be too much for her. To this day, that refrain sometimes rings in my head, as do some of the other things she said repeatedly: "Don't be so dramatic! You're being hysterical!"

I suppose the overriding messages I internalized were *I must not have needs. I no longer matter. I have to be quiet to be tolerated.* Because my mother, in her loneliness, required so much emotional sustenance, and I was a child—a confused, grieving one at that—my default mode network probably also clocked the messages *I have to take care of other people to be loved* and *My suffering is irrelevant.* And because she was my only living parent and there was nowhere else to turn, I also took in the message *No one will help me.* My mother most often expressed approval of me when I set aside my own needs to tend to hers. Then I would hear, "Oh, you are a good daughter!" Or "It's you and me against the world—don't ever forget it!"

At first, it was confusing. My father had always enjoyed hearing what I had to say. He had never deemed me dramatic; rather, he'd encouraged me to be creative, to pen and perform my own playful songs, write my own poems and short stories and recite them for him. When I wrote and illustrated a "book" and gave it to him, he couldn't have been more delighted. This switch in the emotional climate in our home was as confusing as it was isolating.

Looking back, I can see that for my mother, widowed with four children at the age of thirty-nine, the emotional needs or opinions of a twelve-year-old would have seemed entirely secondary to the challenge of figuring out how to just keep that daughter and the rest of her children fed, clothed, safe, and housed. But as a child, I was incapable of taking that perspective. All I knew was I had been delivered into the land of not mattering. So I retreated ever further into myself—taking that message deep within.

Today, having been through my own harrowing experiences as a young parent—there were years when various health complications made me less of a mother than I wanted to be—I feel deep compassion for my mother. What a terrifying time it had to have been for her. I feel admiration, too: With no help from anyone, she went back to school, got a job, and kept a roof over our heads. But the bravery and fortitude and sheer hard work so often required of us in the adult world is unknowable from the vantage point of a child.

And so, as children will, I internalized the message that to be needy was to be bad, damaged, and wholly unlovable. Today, my brain still sometimes spins into what I call my *vortex*, when something occurs that makes me feel ignored, denigrated, or dismissed. This brings up a parade of *mental imagery* and stories about the shame I felt in the past whenever I was put down or criticized by my mother. My thought worms always go back to this central story. *If I have needs or speak up for myself, I am unlovable.* I describe the emotions that are evoked as being like *a ball of dread that I'll be punished or retaliated against*, and the bodily sensations I feel are a sense of lightheadedness and being spaced out (a.k.a. *a space cadet*). A wave of heat comes over me and my whole upper body seems to contract, as if some burning thing has slammed into my chest and bruised me at my core.

In this way, my vortex makes complete sense. It is, in fact, offering me important information about what makes my Inner Defeatist slip into unhealthy rumination in the first place. When I see the connections between my mental imagery, interior emotions, and somatic sensations, and tie it all together, my whole brain lights up with a new awareness: *Oh, here is my old story that if I have needs, I'm not lovable, which fills me with dread, and that fear slams into my solar plexus.* And then it all just . . . starts to dissipate. By regularly practicing MIST, it becomes almost immediately evident to me when these old stories, feelings, and sensations are coming up and commandeering my headspace.

◆ ◆ ◆ ◆

But practicing MIST is not enough, of course. As the British writer China Mieville once wrote, "A trap is only a trap if you don't know about it. If you know about it, it's a challenge." MIST is an exercise in knowing your traps—the traps you are in now, the traps that were set for you in your childhood. Once you know, you can begin to meet the challenge of freeing yourself from them.

III

How to Make a Radically Different Choice

SEVEN

Ballistic Interruption

IF YOU'VE TRIED the MIST Technique and started to decode what your bespoke patterns of rumination have to tell you, well done. The MIST Technique can give you profound insights into your story. But insight alone does not produce lasting change. Once you have a sense of what it's like to escape your mind drama, even briefly, you will also need strategies to help you remain beyond your Inner Defeatist's grasp over the long term. Luckily, there are new neuroscience-based hacks to make this simpler and more doable than ever, and one of them involves talking to yourself—a practice we might call *ballistic interruption.*

Ballistic interrupters help you interrupt and exit ruminating thought patterns so you can engage in more creative thinking and problem-solving. (Just as an aside: In the manufacturing and defense world, a ballistic interrupter is a safety feature that protects defense equipment from exploding during transport. But I think it can also apply to protecting ourselves from our most harmful, self-defeating thought bombs.)

This practice works so well—it can be lightning fast in its effects—because the brain's neuroplasticity makes it highly attentive to verbal signals of redirection. You can use ballistic, or pattern, interrupters to coach your default mode network in a way that effectively wrests it out of its downward spiral. This is crucial if you hope to foster new neural pathways that, over time, translate into new ways of being.

At first, talking to yourself might seem silly. But language that is self-generated by your brain is the language your brain is most likely to pay attention to, which is why when you're mentally berating yourself, you believe so absolutely in the truth of your own negative thoughts. Ballistic interruption messages, which are positive ones instead of negative ones, take advantage of your brain's tendency to believe what you tell it.

Your brain is influenced by the tenor and quality of how you talk to yourself—not unlike the way the music on a radio station playing in the background influences your mood, concentration, and emotions—so if you can find the right words to coax your default mode network into changing its tune, you can bring yourself out of negativity.

Using Ballistic Interrupters

Following are examples of some ballistic interrupters that may give you some ideas about how to talk to yourself. And if they don't resonate with you, you can create your own. Think of them as linguistic hacks that can help you to dispel unhelpful, negative self-beliefs in record time. Or think of them as simple-seeming interventions for complicated people.

The idea here is to find words that land in your psyche so that you feel their visceral power—their weight, import, and authority—in your very bones. Often these are words your brain is not expecting to hear from you. The element of surprise is one of the reasons that these messages are able to interrupt your ruminative narrative so effectively. It's almost as though you've shocked your default mode network into releasing the story it's been holding on to for so long. This is one way to shift your brain's response from hypervigilance to self-regulation.

These pattern interrupters might seem generic at first. That's okay. If you experiment and play with them, you'll eventually land on one that, for you, carries real emotional grit and staying power.

Category One: The Self-Command

These simple self-commands can be an easy way to begin experimenting with ballistic interruption. Here are a few to try when you feel yourself slipping into rumination.

"Cancel that!"

"Delete!"

"Stop it!"

"Nope!"

"Not going there!"

"Let it go!"

"Release!"

"Forget about it!"

"Not helpful!"

"I don't listen to fear-based thoughts!"

"I'm done with thinking about this!"

"I won't even allow this thought in my head!"

"This way of thinking is no longer welcome here!"

"I'm hanging up on you right now! Goodbye and so long!"

"Forget about it! I'm closing this door now!"

"We're not going there!"

My favorite self-command is this: "That's so far outside of the realm of possibility, I'm not even going to consider it!"

This phrase came to me one day when I recalled how I used to say it to my kids when they were young and perseverating on a fear that wasn't real. For instance, if one of them kept asking, "But what if there *are* monsters in my closet?" I'd give them a big hug and say, "That's so far outside the realm of possibility, we're not even going to consider it!" We'd already looked in the closet; they knew there were no monsters hiding there. But it wasn't seeing that really convinced them; it was the certainty of my words that allowed them to let go of their fear and drift off to sleep. In truth, our ruminating mind is no wiser than a child's spinning stories of monsters in the closet.

Category Two: Mantras of Self-Care

Once your early stories take hold—you're a bother, a burden, too needy, dramatic, emotional, loud, opinionated, rambunctious, selfish, chatty, curious—these entrenched beliefs create neural grooves that become harder and harder to get out of the longer you hold on to them. But after a lifetime of negative self-talk, the following pattern interrupters may help you talk to yourself with compassion, reassurance, and kindness, while still embodying the forcefulness of ballistic interruption:

> "I am safe, and it's okay for me to experience all my feelings."

> "I choose to let go of these thoughts, because they don't serve me and I don't need them."

> "I'm good at letting go of my ruminating thoughts, and I choose to do so right now."

> "I know my ruminations are an attempt to think my way out of the situation that's upsetting me, but they are hurting me, not helping me, and it's time to let them go."

"I know these fear-based thoughts no longer serve me."

"I know I am stronger now, and I can handle whatever comes my way."

"I might not like what is happening right now, but I am safe."

"I'm healing from my old way of responding and being."

"I trust this process and what I am learning."

"I am safe and calm, and I know I'll be able to stay that way no matter what."

Category Three: Self-Distancing Talk

For people who resist that kind of self-talk as unconvincing, there's another approach—talk to yourself as if you are an outside observer. This is something we usually do only when we want to scold ourselves ("Ohmigod, Donna, how could you have dropped that bottle of olive oil on the floor? What a klutz!"). But we can also use self-distancing language when we want to reassure ourselves that we are okay. There's actually research to show that when we shift out of "I talk" and refer to ourselves as "you" or by our own name during high-stress moments, we maximize the power of the regulatory effects of self-talk in our brains.

Experimental psychologist Ethan Kross, director of the Emotion & Self-Control Lab at the University of Michigan, researched the effects of self-distancing talk and showed that talking to yourself this way can result in a greater ability to regulate difficult feelings and emotions and put things in perspective.

To understand why this is so, think about how relatively easy it is for you to talk to a friend about his problem and give him good advice, as my friend did when she pointed out that my ruminating about my conflict with the British researcher was getting me nowhere. Addressing yourself in the second person (as "you") is a way of finding enough distance from yourself that you can see your own issues with as much perspective as you can see your friend's, as Kross explains in his book *Chatter.* Not only does self-distancing talk quiet the mind and "shorten the amount of time people spent ruminating," it also lowers stress hormones. For instance, instead of saying, "I can't handle this," tell yourself, "You can handle this."

> "You've got this!"
>
> "You're okay, you're okay."
>
> "You're good at handling difficult feelings, and you'll handle this, too."
>
> "You know how to make good decisions even in difficult situations."
>
> "You know how to take care of yourself. What do you need right now?"

Talking to yourself in the third person, and referring to yourself by your own name, which is known as *illeism,* is something Kross has observed that many famous, successful people do. LeBron James often refers to himself in the third person. Malala Yousafzai uses the third person when speaking about her activism. In a 2015 *New York Times* interview, actress Jennifer Lawrence used self-distancing language to help regulate herself when she became emotional in response to questions during the interview, "O.K., get ahold of yourself, Jennifer. This is not therapy."

Studies looking at the language individuals use when posting on social media have shown that increased use of first-person singular pronouns (*I, me, my*) is associated with a greater likelihood and severity of developing depression. Perhaps this is because first-person pronouns make our experience seem as if whatever difficulty we are experiencing is so personal that it is happening only to us and we are alone in our despair.

Talking to yourself in the tone of a supportive friend who is stepping in to help can interrupt this *I* thinking and can nudge the default mode network out of negative self-talk and self-judgment. And it helps your brain shift from self-critique into self-monitoring mode, which gives you distance from your ruminative thoughts, while having a direct and measurable effect on your neurochemistry.

When I try to do this, I sometimes imagine channeling the voice of my father, grandmother, aunt, or another figure in my life who used a soothing tone with me as a child.

> "Donna, sweetheart, it's okay, you're safe, and everything is going to turn out fine."
>
> "Donna, you've got this, you've done it before, and you can do it again, because you've got everything you need inside you to handle this."
>
> "Donna, you did nothing wrong; there is no need to blame yourself."

I know, I know, this all sounds like motivational fluff. But it's not just positive psychology, it's neurobiology: The way you speak to yourself changes not only how you feel in the moment but the way your default mode network habitually wires itself.

Create Your Own Bespoke Ballistic Interrupter

For many people, it's important to create their own ballistic interrupter, one that is tailored very specifically to the narratives that keep repeating in their heads. For Sam, using ballistic interrupters during difficult conversations with his med school adviser has helped him to step back, before he plummets into the dark mental pit of rumination. Recently, his adviser told him that a fellow med student's performance in the operating room had been "excellent, exceptional, exactly what we're looking for here." When he heard these words, Sam said he felt "the old gravitational pull of my mind drama. I started to fall into thought spirals about how I was letting my professor down, while also worrying that he was taking a jab at me because I wasn't as good as his prize mentee, and maybe I wasn't 'what we're looking for.'"

Sam ballistically interrupted himself by (silently) telling himself: "Cut it out, wise guy. I see what you're trying to do here! Not today you don't!" This bespoke ballistic interrupter shut down his mind drama before it could get out of control. At other times, Sam personifies the bully in his head and turns his Inner Defeatist's critiques back against *it*, using the same language it's using against *him*. "If I catch myself telling myself, 'You're never good enough. You suck,' I tell my Inner Defeatist, 'No, you're the one who sucks! You suck for trying to keep me from succeeding at the things I want to do in life! Stop it!'"

Even more impressive is that this practice has yielded some deeper insights that build upon those he gleaned from MIST, Sam tells me. "When I stop the story, I get clarity on what's going on for me, what really matters." This includes the awareness that "my adviser can be a class A jerk, sure. But he's not my real problem. One day when I was obsessing about whether I should pursue surgery, as he wants me to, I used a ballistic interrupter that came into my head out of nowhere: 'What do you think you're doing? You don't want to be a surgeon, you never did, and that's that!'" And suddenly that allowed Sam to make connections that he never saw before. Sam's father was a well-known surgeon, he explains, "so I kept leaning in that direction because I wanted not only my professor's approval but my dad's. I guess some part of me knows, deep down, that I've always believed that if I could only get my dad's approval, that would be as close as I'll ever get to feeling he loves me."

With the help of his interrupter, everything became so much simpler: He did not want to be a surgeon. Now all he had to do was figure out what he did want to be.

◆ ◆ ◆ ◆

Sometimes, like Sam, we know exactly what's triggering our mind drama—in his case, his conflicts with his professor. But sometimes, we don't know the underlying reason we find ourselves mired, once again, in self-deprecation. For my friend Virginia, "the trip wire into a downward thought spiral can be the tiniest, merest echo of feelings that reignite those early, awful feelings of unworthiness—that I'm being humiliated, invalidated, or put down. But sometimes I'm not sure what, precisely, elicited these feelings in me. I just know I'm feeling them again."

Using ballistic interruption helps Virginia not only stop this mind-steal but data-mine it for insight as to what's given rise to her Inner Defeatist. First, Virginia uses the MIST Technique to reorient herself: "Oh, here's that old denigrated, I'm-not-respected, debilitating feeling of worthlessness." Once she realizes she's "circling the drain again," Virginia invokes her bespoke ballistic interrupter: "No, no, no, no, no you don't! Wait a minute!" This simple verbal stop sign allows her to look more deeply at what's going on inside. "I look back at the catalog of all that mental imagery coursing through my mind to make sure I'm being clear about what's bugging me. Once I see, 'Oh! It was *that* conversation with so-and-so, when they said *that* to me,' I try to distinguish between criticisms that might be valid and teach me something, and those that are not valid, which I must wholeheartedly reject." Then—and I love this—Virginia uses a second ballistic interrupter to address her critics this way: "Who said *you* get to decide my future? Who appointed *you* the boss of me? I reject you and everything you're saying."

Once she's done this, Virginia is able to back out from behind enemy lines—that war zone where she's always worrying about what other people think of her. "I can tell myself, 'Okay, okay, I can listen to what other people have to say, some of their comments might even be helpful, but I have to ignore the ones that aren't. I couldn't do that with my father. But I can do that now.'"

Finally, as a highly visual person, Virginia has another shortcut she uses to ballistically interrupt her thinking—a strategy I plan to borrow for myself. "I imagine painting the word *rumination* on a canvas. Then I use paint to cross out the letter *m* so the word becomes *ruination.* That reminds me I don't have to ruin my day—or week—with rumination."

Ada, who works in set design and film, has put her own visual spin on the concept of ballistic interruption. "As soon as I start worrying that I said the wrong thing to Allie—something which falls into the bad-mom domain of being just like my mom—I imagine that the scene replaying in my head is playing on a computer screen and I'm using movie-editing software. I hear my fingers click across the computer keys as I delete, delete, delete those thoughts. Then I sit back and watch the screen fade to black." After that, Ada adds in this mantra: "That may be someone else's story, but it's not *my* story."

Ada has one more trick, which I, too, find helpful. "When I'm perseverating over a conversation I had with Carl, or a conversation with a friend isn't sitting right with me, or someone hasn't texted me back and I'm wondering why, it helps to remind myself that I can never truly know what others are thinking or feeling." Ada's ballistic interrupter for these situations is to tell herself, " 'They don't know, and I don't know.' It's a very freeing message. It opens me up to more compassion, for them, for me."

That small moment of curiosity, especially when directed toward her husband, and how he might be feeling unsure, or suffering in some way, changes what happens next. When a feeling of compassion for Carl comes over her, it leads Ada to make an effort to see what might be causing him distress. "I can see how hard it has been for him these past few years, as I've gotten busier with my work, and he's more or less retired, that there isn't that much happening for him right now. I understand he wants to be useful. He wants to be needed; he's worried about losing his voice and his power." It's not all smooth sailing, and, as in any marriage, there is more work to be done, but recently, there are no more butter knives being wielded in the kitchen. "For the past few years, there's often been this live wire of contention buzzing between my husband and me whenever we're in the same room. You can feel it; I think my daughter can feel it. But by trying to see things from his point of view, I've let go of a lot of my resentment. I can be firm with him about his micromanaging, but I don't seethe with anger all the time. So a lot of the old, habitual tension is gone."

Because I take such solace in nature, and this is where I found solace as a child after the death of my father, my favorite self-made ballistic interrupter is to simply repeat to myself, over and over, "Seeing beauty, seeing light, seeing beauty, seeing light." This happened for me organically one day when I was out for a walk on a perfectly lovely late afternoon, around the golden hour. I'd caught myself ruminating and mired in uncertainty about events in the news, worrisome events I had zero control over. As I was trying to interrupt those thought spirals, the sun broke through the clouds. Light angled over the fields, suddenly illuminating the antlers of a young five-point buck, startling him. He looked up at me as if to inquire what was happening. We locked eyes for a split second. The light shifted, playing over the sycamore trees in our field, turning the bare areas where the bark had peeled off to a bright, ethereal white. The tips of the oak trees, still touched by rainwater from a brief afternoon shower, lit up like shards of fire.

I suddenly heard myself uttering, *I'm seeing beauty everywhere.* And that felt so good, like such a welcome balm, I added, *I'm seeing beauty and light everywhere.* I just kept rotating those words in my mouth, *Seeing beauty, seeing light.* And that became a softball ballistic interrupter that continues to hold great power for me whenever my darker thoughts threaten to abscond with me. It has an added benefit: The more I notice the beauty, the light, around me, the more I see. (This is thanks to a filtering system in our brains, known as the *reticular activating system.*) Recently, I added two more words to my mantra: *Seeing beauty, seeing light, seeing love.* When I use this mantra while with my family and friends, the words flood me with warmth, while making me more emotionally present, more in love with my life and all its precious offerings. It's like creating a mental snow globe, one that shimmers in my mind, only I am both looking at the enchanted scene and living inside it.

Whichever tool you use for ballistic interruption, by taking this step, you're developing a skill that will help you hone your internal locus of control for managing your rumination. The more you use these positive missives to help redirect and rewire your default mode network, the less and less likely you are to revert to the negative messages that keep you locked in your mind drama.

EIGHT

Body-State Breakers

"SOMETIMES I'M SO caught up in my thoughts, I feel like my head is floating outside my body," Paola says, laughing in a slightly self-deprecating way. "It's like I've uploaded my brain to the cloud, and I only exist there." This disembodied state, she adds, "fuels this low-grade feeling of hypervigilance it's hard to give words to." Paola's mind is on her body because her internist had recently told her, after he did an exam and ran some blood work, that she had high blood pressure, high cholesterol, and an underactive thyroid. Her doctor put her on a thyroid medication and said if her cholesterol levels climb any further, she will need to consider going on statins. Paola feels she's "getting all these fun conditions in my late fifties, before most of my friends." Her lower back is also bothering her. "It's an old injury from a trip Will and I did years ago, when we were spelunking." The rope attached to Paola's harness got wet and she slipped a few feet. "My back slammed into a rock."

She can't help but wonder if some of her medical issues are tied up with "all the uncertainty I've been feeling in my marriage," she tells me. The fun, jokey, sexy, competitive communication style Will has always had, which once seemed to her to be witty if a bit sophomoric, "is becoming more and more unbearable. It seems so self-involved, narcissistic. Like he can get away with being controlling or quipping or 'ha ha funny' little put-downs because, well, he's just a guy being a guy." What Paola used to tolerate now feels—and is—unacceptable.

As Paola speaks, I'm reminded of a line from Lorrie Moore's book *Anagrams.* A husband says something quite hurtful to his wife—in Moore's story, it's about the unlikelihood of his being faithful. The wife thinks, "I couldn't believe my ears. Was this the difference between men and women? That women could never believe their ears?"

Paola seems to experience this wave of disbelief a lot with Will, given the things that come out of his mouth. She tells me about a time a year or so ago when she and Will were in the car on the way to visit a friend who lived several hours away, and Paola was driving. She was distracted and missed one of their exits on the highway. She got back on the highway and all was fine. Then, a few hours later, when they were about an hour from their friend's house, she turned on the wrong street. A car pulled up in the lane beside them and came to a stop a bit ahead of their car. The car's license plate read: NITWIT.

Will laughed out loud and said, "I should get you that license plate!"

"This fierce, hot wind blew right into me," Paola recalls. "My whole body, the whole core of me, stung as if I'd been buried by a sandstorm. I couldn't speak. I couldn't believe he would say that. I could barely breathe I was so angry."

The rest of the drive was "deadly silent," Paola recounts. "Will didn't say a word. He knew he'd fucked up again, and he was too immature to apologize. Meanwhile, I was fuming, my heart was thumping. I felt this punch; my gut hurt as if I'd eaten something rotten." For years, after such incidents, Paola would write them down in her "Will Book," a journal in which she listed the "little bitty shitty" things he said. Why catalog them? "I always thought if I decided to leave, it would be good to have, so I could remind myself why I had left him, in case I second-guessed myself."

But more recently, since getting better at discerning what tips her into rumination and why, and "realizing that my altered state of thinking will only make things worse," Paola takes a different, emotionally healthier approach. It combines a new personal rumination code with a ballistic interrupter. Her personal rumination code is this: *"Here is my old picture book of how people diminish me, which hits my nervous system like a hot wind so I can't breathe."* And when she's angry with Will, she uses a ballistic interrupter she has developed to calm herself down. Paola channels the soothing voice of her grandmother, who often consoled her as a child: "I hear you, Paola. This hurts—of course it does. Anyone would feel that way. What do you need me to do right now to take care of you?"

Usually, Paola says, "The answer that comes is that I need to put my head back on my body, pay attention to what I'm feeling in my body. When I try to do that, I realize I'm not really breathing. I'm so contracted and curled up inside myself it hurts. It's like I'm stuck in this hypervigilance, waiting for that hot wind to plow into me again."

As Paola listens to this burgeoning voice within, her self-inquiry is starting to redirect her default mode network's Inner Defeatist–run operating system. Still, it's hard for Paola to figure out what her body needs to feel safe again. "My body is lagging behind the changes I'm making. My thoughts are less seething and toxic, but my body still feels tense to the point that it's hard for me to get my body to agree with my head that everything will be okay, we've got this."

As Paola has intuited, even though she doesn't yet know what to do about it, the doorway to a sense of internal well-being is often through the very thing that you always carry with you: your body. (Bessel van der Kolk put it best in his book title *The Body Keeps the Score.*) Once we pay attention to how our pain and fear show up in our bodies, something shifts.

The Physical Fallout from Your Thought Spirals

One reason why rumination takes such a toll on your body is that when you habitually replay negative storylines in which you are the starring actor, narrator, and director, your brain can't tell the difference between stressful events unfolding in real time and imaginary or remembered events. Each time your mind relives a stressful scenario, your body relives it, too, as if that bad thing were still happening. The more often you put it on rewind, the worse it is for your physical body, and the more you inflict upon yourself what researchers call *secondary harm.*

Given Paola's recent health issues and her growing sense of mortality, she is determined to "graduate into the courage to be disliked." She's not there yet, but I can hear in her voice that something is shifting inside her—something as powerful as it is empowering. Psychologist John Gottman, PhD, who studies relationships, has examined the physical effects of what happens when we are dismissed or humiliated and fear speaking up for ourselves. "There is absolutely no such thing as constructive criticism," he argues. "Anybody who gets put down, insulted, treated with sarcasm or insults or mockery, actually gets more physically ill over time." In his book *When the Body Says No,* Gabor Maté shares the stark study of two thousand women over ten years that found that unhappily married women who didn't express their feelings were four times more likely to die compared to those who did express how they felt—even while remaining unhappily married. It's as if the body senses the struggle to create boundaries. If we can't say no, our bodies will. Seen in this light, Paola's decision to speak up for herself in those vulnerable moments when she feels dismissed or ridiculed—rather than turning inward and ruminating—is nothing short of courageous.

On the cellular level, the longer you ruminate, the more these biological ill effects literally travel deep into your biology. Neuroscientists recently mapped out precisely how psychological stress can trigger a cascade of stress hormones and chemicals that reach all the way into your cell's energy centers, known as *mitochondria.* Mitochondria are tiny but have a mighty job. Like an overhead dimmer switch on a chandelier, mitochondria power your mental capacity and physical stamina up or down. You can thank your mitochondria for how energetic your body and mind feel throughout the day. As incredible as it might sound, all the mitochondria in your brain, bones, tissues, and organs are always communicating with one another in one big, chatty network. And one of the things that they are chattering about revolves around this question: How safe are you right now?

Our brains and bodies are always listening for signs of danger while simultaneously seeking signals of safety. To gauge how safe you are, your body uses a process known as *neuroception* to gather information from all your senses. But here's the problem: The human nervous system evolved long before conscious, logical thought, so it maneuvers within a significant margin of error when it comes to assessing how much danger you face.

According to DeLisa Fairweather, professor of medicine and immunologist at the Mayo Clinic in Jacksonville, Florida, "Mitochondria are always alerting us to danger." When the incoming message is that you are not safe, mitochondria sense and respond to these signals, passing along the message—"Incoming threat!"—like a telegram being handed off from one cell to the next. (Mitochondria do this, Fairweather explains, through something called *extracellular vesicles*, which are like tiny bubbles that travel throughout your body, relaying biological instructions between cells.) When your brain clocks a threat—your coworker rolls his eyes after you share your idea at a staff meeting, your parent makes that old, cutting remark about you again at the dinner table, your partner lets out a derisive laugh after you vulnerably share your feelings—these missives that you are being devalued, you don't matter, get relayed through your mitochondria, giving each little cell an ignition spark of fear at its center.

And yes, you guessed it, these threat messages can be initiated by the words you silently mutter to yourself inside your head. The longer this threat sensation steals through your body, the more cortisol and adrenaline levels spike and your blood pressure and heart rate rise. Your cells respond as if you're in physical danger (some researchers call this process the *cell danger response*) and send SOS messages to other cells, triggering genes to turn on defenses that eventually put you at risk for higher levels of physical inflammation and disease. It's a well-meant but misguided attempt to protect you.

This can be especially true when your pattern of rumination began in childhood. In one 2020 international study using brain scans, researchers found when individuals who'd experienced childhood adversity faced periods of stress in adulthood, their levels of inflammatory chemicals and hormones rose significantly faster and higher than among those without a history of childhood adversity. Those who dealt with early adversity also showed more rumination-associated activity in the brain. In other words, those of us who faced chronic childhood stress have a lower set point at which these stress-response patterns get flipped on. Researchers call this *stress sensitization:* You react to stress more quickly and with more oomph, and it's harder to turn that stress response off after the stressor has passed.

That's the alarming news. But here's the extremely good news: This physical cascade is as malleable as our thoughts. Even when we are caught up in a state of brooding rumination, and messages fly from cell to cell spreading their dark missives about imminent threats, we still have tremendous power to start anew and set ourselves on a very different path. The longer we've been caught in a pattern of turning on ourselves, the longer it might take. But it is all reversible. This is true, no matter what your story might be.

We just have to work with our bodies, alongside our thoughts.

When we consider what this new research tells us about the possibility for change, I think our work here, to interrupt the threat signals we send ourselves, is one of the greatest acts of self-love we can perform.

For me, this is, admittedly, the hardest step in my effort to quell my rumination habit, perhaps because, given my history of health issues, it's challenging for me to truly believe my body can ever be a safe place to reside. But cultivating a feeling of safety within my body is also the thing that is most likely to save me. It might save you, too.

In one of my meetings with neuroscientist Mark Trullinger, he shed a new and illuminating light on why somatic experiencing, or being present with what my body is feeling, might be so challenging for me. Trullinger hooked me up to electrodes, which register brain waves, while we chatted. He asked me to talk about my "medical trauma," including my first hospitalization for von Willebrand disease, a rare bleeding disorder, at the age of five. We touched on the treatments I'd undergone for that and other blood disorders, which sometimes required receiving coagulants, and intravenous infusions of other people's blood parts, to assist my immune system in healing. He asked me brief questions about the heart procedures I'd undergone and the periods of paralysis I'd faced due to a neurological autoimmune disease, as well as other memories I rarely dredge up, because remembering them makes my heart pound in fear it might all happen again, so I'm not even going to write them down here. Just by writing these words, dear reader, my heart is thundering.

My lifelong approach has been that if I don't speak or think about these events in my life, they aren't relevant, and my life can go on as it is. Crisis-free. Nothing to see here.

But after our talk, Trullinger showed me something that made me question my suppress-it-to-survive-it approach.

He turned his computer around to show me what my brain had looked like when I'd delved into my medical history. "This is where you process your somatic sensations," he told me. He pointed to the area of my default mode network, the parietal lobe, which plays a role in generating and registering physical, bodily sensations. He zeroed in on an area on the right side of my brain. It was going haywire.

My brain was still hooked up to Trullinger's computer via silver electrodes and a web of black wires as I stared at the huge spike in my brain wave activity.

"Wow," Trullinger said, his tone surprised. "When I just said the word *somatic*, your heart rate spiked again, and your brain waves responded in a way we see in individuals who are feeling extremely traumatized and dysregulated, and caught in a fight-or-flight response."

"Why would I go into fight or flight at the mention of the word *somatic*?" I ask.

"Well, *somatic* is a word that's often used to discount and negate the validity of women's experiences. Especially in our medical system. And in your lifetime, that's probably happened to you."

"Oh. Right," I say, letting this revelation wash over me. "Right."

"It's little wonder your brain jumps at the mere mention of the word. For you, the word *somatic* signals danger—the danger of being invalidated as a woman, as a patient."

How many times had the medical establishment treated me—and so many other women—as if I were making things up? When I was five, and in the hospital for a tonsillectomy, I hadn't yet been diagnosed with von Willebrand disease, and during surgery, I hemorrhaged badly. I spent a week in the hospital, recovering, and can still recall vomiting blood, my mouth being packed and repacked with ice and gauze until the sutures at last began to heal. Soon after that, I did receive the diagnosis, which, in turn, led to my family becoming part of a decades-long hematological study at Johns Hopkins. My father, one of my older brothers, my grandmother, and I all had this congenital bleeding disorder. But even with this diagnosis, it didn't keep doctors from thinking I was being dramatic—hormonal—when, at the age of fifteen, I complained of having extremely long and heavy periods that could last three weeks. It would take decades before a doctor told me these menstrual issues were not uncommon in female patients with von Willebrand disease.

Sometimes this feeling of being dismissed and diminished affects things that happen in my work life, as was the case with the British researcher—another reason I probably responded so strongly to that incident. But after doing thousands of interviews in my life, I know many, if not most, women carry their own stories of being gaslit about their bodies and feeling diminished by experts within our healthcare system who don't believe them. What woman hasn't found herself being mansplained to about her own body? Nothing new here.

I pulled myself, with difficulty, out of these mental movies about these and other episodes in my health history—the past scenes flicking through my head, zipping by as if on fast-forward—and looked up at Trullinger, who was now mid-sentence.

"—and because of these experiences, you have discounted the validity of your own story," he was saying. "Somatic exercises will help you with this."

As I learned when researching these exercises, Thomas Louis Hanna, PhD, a philosophy professor and movement specialist, first coined the term *somatics* in 1976. Hanna, who also studied neurology, developed the idea that all life experiences lead to physical patterns we hold in the body. Hanna explains this concept, which he calls Sensory Motor Amnesia (SMA), in a way I find helpful. When we face adversity, or trauma, the communication between our brains, muscles, and nervous systems becomes impaired. We hold extra tension in our bodies, but that chronic tension becomes so habituated, so normal for us, that our brains are no longer aware we're doing this. Our muscles stay contracted, but outside of our conscious awareness. And herein lies a problem. If you don't notice that tension, you can't release it. Your brain can't direct your muscles to relax.

The longer our stress physiology has been stuck on overdrive—and I'd been stuck for a very long time—the more helpful it may be to employ somatic practices that can signal to our bodies that have fled the danger our brains keep telling us to watch out for. *We are okay, we are safe,* these practices tell us. As you learn and practice the following somatic skills, you'll help stimulate and free up the vitality that is stored deep in your mitochondria, which constitutes your inexhaustible life force.

Micro-Moment Body-State Breakers

What follows are science-based actionable skills to send messages to your body and brain that will enhance your feeling of being safe. Instead of muscling through, pushing on, or trying to make something inside "go away," these practices help you support yourself even as you have difficult feelings, emotions, or sensations. As you practice these, think of them as a set of circuit breaker switches in the electrical panel in your brain that you can use anytime, with immediate effect. (One note here: When trauma has been severe, you may need more somatic coaching with a practitioner. For more on this, see chapter 12, "When You Need More Help.")

These body-state breakers are not a one-and-done. This is a lifestyle practice. Your body has been right here with you, responding to your most difficult life experiences in real time. According to Paul Conti, MD, a former Stanford and Harvard psychiatrist, most if not all of us have "had major past stressors in our lives or adversity that is stored in our nervous system, modifying our brain and neural circuitry," including the function of our default mode network. These practices will help to reawaken your sense of "you" by bringing your body and mind back into your current experience, emotionally and energetically. We might even say *mitochondrially.*

Some of the practices I share here are thousands of years old and are taught in various permutations by experts, coaches, and therapists worldwide. Anyone who practices mind-body techniques, including yoga, mindfulness, and breath practices, will see similarities. The versions I describe are the ones I've found to be the best companion practices to MIST, and the most helpful in enabling you to exit self-deprecating, anxious-making overthinking, while anchoring you in a profound feeling of safety. They take only a few minutes to practice and will help you to release all that was never yours to carry.

The Body-State Breaker Sigh

The average person sighs twelve times an hour. Often, we don't even notice we're doing it. We might be bored, frustrated, or holding back a strong emotion. But we can make conscious use of sighing to exit a state of rumination and thereby alleviate the physiological arousal that so often accompanies our ruminations. Stanford neuroscientist Andrew Huberman found in a study of 111 individuals that "cyclic sighing" signals the respiratory system it's okay to calm down, you're safe, it's okay to relax. Individuals who practiced cyclic sighing every day for a month experienced reduced anxiety and increased positive emotions—more so than those who practiced mindful meditation. Here is a version of cyclical sighing—also known as the *physiological sigh*—which I have added to and adapted and teach in my workshops. In this version, I combine sighing with a microburst of movement.

- Stand up. (Or, if you can't stand, you can also practice this while sitting.)
- Close your lips and take in a full, slow inhale as you raise your arms overhead.
- As you keep your arms up, open and tightly close your fists, and vigorously shake out your hands.
- Exhale, relax your breath, while still keeping your arms overhead.
- Inhale again and pause for just a second while holding that breath.
- Now, take in a second inhale, deepening your inhalation so that it fills your whole belly, chest, all the way up to your collarbone.

- Let out a long exhalation from your mouth, sighing loudly and dramatically, letting it all go.
- Allow your arms to gently float down to your sides.
- Repeat this for five minutes.
- How do you feel?

Sixty-Second Self-Soother

This is a powerful technique—rooted in neuroscience—that centers on the vagus nerve, the body's largest nerve and a key player in regulating our emotional and physical states. When we activate the vagus nerve, we're not just calming ourselves, we're leveraging a built-in system for emotional regulation. Stimulating the vagus nerve can help us shift out of rumination and into a state of calm, often in just a few minutes. The exercise I'm sharing is adapted from a technique taught to me by trauma therapist Marti Glenn, PhD. It's designed to activate your nervous system's self-soothing capacities in ways that lower your stress response in two minutes.

- Close your eyes. Inhale. Exhale.
- Place a hand on each ear. Softly grip your ears and gently pull on the outer part of both earlobes as if stretching or widening them to the side. (Think Dumbo ears.) Start at the top of your earlobes and do this all the way down to the bottom of them (to the lower lobe, where you might place an earring).
- Gently put your middle finger inside the inner shell-like part of your right ear, softly circle it around, then gently pull down on that earlobe and hold for ten seconds.
- Repeat this sequence in your left ear. You might yawn. (This is your vagal system relaxing!)

- Slide your hands down to gently stroke your chin, the way someone who loved you as a child might have.
- Gently stroke your collarbone.
- Slide your hands over your heart and apply light pressure there.
- See if any positive self-soothing phrases come to mind: "I am safe." "I am loved." "I belong."
- Open your eyes. See if you feel any different.

The Rosenberg Technique

The Rosenberg Technique for relaxation was created by Stanley Rosenberg, who referred to it as the "Basic Exercise." It involves gazing peripherally to both right and left, and it's a powerful way to send your brain the message that you are safe. The reason for this is that across evolutionary time, we only looked peripherally when we were sure nothing bad was about to happen to us, and could afford to allow our gaze to wander. Rosenberg's technique is a quick and potent way to tell your body you're safe, regardless of your spiraling thoughts—and it is a personal favorite of mine. This technique also increases blood flow to the brain stem and supports healthy vagal nerve function, leading to an overall sense of relaxation and well-being.

- Sit or lie down comfortably.
- Interlock your fingers behind your head.
- While keeping your neck and head facing forward, look to the right with your eyes only.
- Hold your gaze there for thirty seconds to a minute, or until you spontaneously yawn or swallow.
- Return to a neutral position with your head and eyes facing straight ahead.

- Repeat this process, this time looking to the left.
- Keep alternating between right and left for several repetitions.
- Enjoy the big yawns this elicits!

Instant Safe Haven

In this exercise, which is the most popular one I teach in my workshops, I am adapting a technique known as Havening, developed by physicians Steven Ruden and Ronald Ruden, and combining it with the practice of ballistic interruption, and with Voo Breath, a breathing technique developed by Peter Levine, PhD, who has pioneered a wide range of somatic body-oriented approaches to healing trauma and other stress-related disorders.

The Havening technique uses gentle stroking of the arms, face, or palms to stimulate what are known as C-tactile fibers in your skin. These sensory fibers, when stimulated, release neurochemicals like serotonin and oxytocin, which promote emotional regulation and calm. Our hands and arms are full of nerves, which are particularly responsive to soft, loving touch, which makes sense since when we are young, we reach up to adults, hoping to be seen, comforted, and held.

The Voo Breath helps bring us out of a state of fear or hypervigilance and tones the vagus nerve. Combining these techniques in the manner below has become my go-to when I need a quick exit from my mind drama.

- Place one palm on your forehead, the other over your heart.
- Imagine you are being comforted by someone with whom you feel safe and seen and valued.
- Move your hands to your chin and hold and stroke it, the way a loving parent might.

- Now, begin to repeatedly slide your hands down your arms, from the top of your shoulders down to the backs of your hands.
- Take a deeper breath in through your nose.
- Exhale through your mouth slowly while making a *voo* sound—the deep sound that a foghorn makes. Focus on the vibration rising in your throat.
- Continue to stroke your arms while making the *voo* sound with each exhale.
- As you gently stroke your arms, ask yourself what positive self-soothing phrases you most long to hear and feel. These might be: "I belong here." "I believe in myself." "I am safe." "I am loved." "I matter."
- As you continue to stroke your arms, on each exhale, repeat whatever phrase feels most emotionally comforting to you in a deep vibrational tone (think of monks chanting in a monastery; that's the vibrational sound you're going for). Notice the vibration in your throat and chest.
- Continue to speak your self-soothing phrase(s) out loud with every exhale.
- Add this step for extra credit: As you chant each exhale, speak these same words while referring to yourself using your own name: "Jane, you belong here." "Paul, you are safe." "Amy, you matter." (For me—perhaps because of my history of medical trauma—this is often, simply, "Donna, you are safe, you are safe, you are safe.") As discussed earlier, self-distancing messaging can be a particularly powerful way of communicating with your default mode network.
- Keep stroking your arms and repeating your message until you feel the words you're chanting resonate inside every cell.

- Repeat this cycle for several minutes.
- Notice how it stimulates a sense of calm.

Roaring Breath (a.k.a. Lion's Roar)

This is a technique taught and used by yogis around the world. (On that note, yoga is a great body-state breaker. The more yoga, the better! But here we're looking for fast strategies, things you can do in five minutes or less, for an immediate release from our mind drama.)

- Take in a breath to the count of four.
- Hold your breath to the count of seven. As you hold your breath, clench your fists and tighten your chest, stomach, arms, and face.
- Exhale for a count of eight as forcefully as you can, with your tongue sticking out and your mouth hanging open, as you make a huge roaring sound.
- Repeat and continue for three to five minutes.

"How Am I Really Feeling?"

Georgie Oldfield, a physical therapist and founder of SIRPA, the Stress Illness Recovery Practitioners' Association, taught me this powerful exercise to help me feel safe in my body even when I am experiencing unwelcome sensations that spark health-anxiety-led rumination. This cathartic technique is unique in that the physical, somatic release (which signals to our bodies that we are safe) is reached through touching into the underlying feelings of danger that are causing that physical tension. As we do, we build up our tolerance for feeling difficult emotions—the very ones our rumination habit is trying to suppress.

- Lie down and scan your body, gently noticing any tightness or pain or sensation that arises.

- Breathe in deeply, noticing if that area feels tight, or hot, or whatever words accurately describe it.
- Repeat "I'm safe" every now and again as you allow yourself to feel your body's sensations.
- Imagine your child self, cuddled up next to you, snuggling up against you, as you hold her close.
- Ask that child self how she's doing, using your first name (e.g., "Donna, how are you really feeling?" or "Donna, what's really going on here?").
- Notice what arises. For many people, it brings up tears. This is often the case for me when I use this technique.
- Now ask yourself, "What's causing the pain/tightness/sensation?" or "What's causing this pain to persist?" or "What is this pain really trying to tell me?"
- Often, something will come to you that helps you to realize your pain or physical tension is trying to tell you something. Usually, it is trying to alert you that there is something going on in your life that is bringing up feelings you're suppressing or aren't dealing with very well.
- Now, ask yourself, "What can I learn from this?" This might mean accepting that whatever is happening is something you can't control. It might mean setting more boundaries with difficult people, or setting aside more time for yourself.
- Ask yourself, "Can I release this?" See what happens. For me, my muscles relax almost instantaneously.
- Ask yourself if you can accept things as they are, and if not, what first steps you might be able to take to make some changes—always being gentle with your expectations for yourself.

I've used this technique many times and been surprised by its power. Once it culminated in my sobbing with grief over various losses in my life and in the lives of loved ones. It felt overwhelming, but also good.

"What can I learn from this?" I asked when I was finally able to find my breath.

The answer was so simple when it came: "It's okay to lie down and have a good cry. We should do this more often."

The Japanese have a term for this experience, this catharsis—*rui katsu*, or "tear seeking"—a full emotional release through which we feel renewed.

I'd had a *rui katsu*. I'd been able to sense my rumination dissipating and finally ending. And I did indeed feel renewed.

Rapid Rescue Muscle Relaxing

Many, many years ago, when I was a senior in college, I signed up for a course in stress reduction to fulfill one of my physical education requirements. A few dozen students were in the class, and to begin, we all lay down on the floor. The teacher started each class with a classic squeeze-and-release exercise. (I confess, it was so relaxing that most of us were snoring on the floor of the gym five minutes into class—the prof didn't seem to mind.) To this day, I still use this technique to quickly exit any mind-drama-induced tension. I often do it right before falling asleep, and (when I can remember to do it) I also do it while I'm at my desk if I'm stuck in a gnarly writing problem. I choose it again and again because it reliably works.

There are a thousand versions of muscle relaxation, or "tense-and-release" exercises—even the military has its own version to help soldiers relax in the field—but here is how I practice it for maximum results:

- Slowly breathe in through your nose to the count of five as you squeeze and contract your hands, making them into tight fists. Hold your breath to the count of four as you continue to squeeze your fists as tightly as you can (within your comfort range). Then, breathe out of your mouth to the count of eight, letting out a big, exaggerated whooshing sound as you release all the tension in your hands. Notice the feeling of relaxation spreading from your wrists down to your fingertips.

- Next begin to focus on your arms and shoulders. Breathe in to the count of five as you gently tense the muscles of your arms and raise your shoulders up toward your ears. Continue to squeeze these muscles as you hold this breath to the count of four. Now release, breathing out of your mouth to the count of eight, letting out a big, whooshing sound. Notice the feeling of relaxation flowing down through your shoulders and arms.
- Next bring your attention to your face. Begin by counting to five as you gently tense the muscles of your forehead. You can do this by wrinkling it into a deep, unhappy, "ugh" frown. Hold this to the count of four. Breathe out to the count of eight, letting out an exaggerated whoosh, and completely let go. Feel the tension leaving your forehead.
- Now, tense your cheeks and jaw. You can do this by smiling extra widely. Breathe in to the count of five as you make an exaggerated "clown face" smile. Count to four as you hold this breath and your expression. Release as you exhale to the count of eight with a big, whooshing sound. Notice the feeling of relaxation coming over your face.
- Move your attention to your back. Breathe in to the count of five as you squeeze and contract the muscles in your back by arching your back up and away from the floor or chair, bringing your shoulder blades together behind you (if comfortable). Count to four as you hold this breath and this position. Release your breath to the

count of eight, letting go with a big, whooshing sound. Enjoy the growing feeling of relaxation.

- Move your attention to your buttocks, pelvic floor, and thighs. Breathe in to the count of five as you squeeze the muscles in your buttocks by pressing them together and tightening your thighs. Add in a Kegel (contracting your pelvic floor and perineum). Hold this breath and contraction to the count of four. Now breathe out to the count of eight with a whooshing sound, completely releasing and letting go. Wriggle your hips as you let this newfound relaxation wash over you.
- Move your attention to your feet. Breathe in to the count of five as you flex your feet and tighten your calves. Count to four as you hold this breath and contraction. Release, exhaling to the count of eight, letting out a full exhalation in a whooshing sound. Now repeat this sequence, only this time, contract your feet by curling your toes instead of flexing them.
- Now, squeeze and contract all the parts of your body for five seconds, before holding for four seconds and letting go with the same eight-second exhalation and whooshing sound. As you do so, picture a light descending from your crown and filling your whole body. Feel it travel down your spine, down your legs, and into the earth that holds you. Relax.
- Do a quick scan through your body to see if there is any residual tension. If you sense any tension at all, simply talk to it, and cajole it into relaxing by saying, "Let it go."
- Notice how you feel. Has anything lifted?

Check the Mirror—and Express the Opposite of What You See

When we're lost in mind drama, our faces show it. You can't hide your ruminative state, not even from your own eyes. Muscles in your jaw tense, your eyes (and eyelids) narrow, your nostrils tighten (or flare), and the muscles around your mouth contract, pulling the corners of your mouth down. For most of us, seeing what we look like when we're spinning stories, judging ourselves, and judging others is not pleasant. Have you ever known that feeling of walking down the street and catching sight of your face—your "at rest" expression—in a store window and thinking, *Wow, is that me?* That's because our faces at rest are often ruminating faces. None of us like the worn-down way we look when we're swept up in thoughts we can't let go of.

So here's a ten-second rescue. When you catch yourself ruminating, go look in a mirror, or take a selfie. Really look at your face, your expression. Take in your narrowed, tight features, the downturned arc of your lips. Now, do the opposite with your face. Start by smiling with your eyes—when you shift the muscles around your eyes, the rest of your facial muscles will follow. Really lean into this experimentation as if you were an improv actor: Add in happy laughter, gestures of gladness and surprise as if greeting your happy self for the first time. Experiment with expressions and gestures until you embody someone who has happily moved beyond your cyclic mind stories. What does that version of you look and feel like? What does she think about? How does she walk, talk, laugh, and smile? Move through the room (or wherever you are) with your joy face and your happy movements for a few minutes and welcome the more jubilant sensations and thoughts that brings. (One caveat here: When I am teaching workshops, I've seen that for some people, when doing this exercise, laughter turns to tears. If that happens to you, that's okay! Tears are good, too! Whatever comes up for you is the thing you need to express and release.)

These body-state breakers have a tremendous payoff: They decrease the amount of time you spend ruminating. By doing these practices, you interrupt the bidirectional feedback loop from body to brain, brain to body, that tells you to be on the alert in the face of danger. You can meet your ramped-up stress response with somatic-level messages of safety, calm, and release. And that, my friends, is another path to finding freedom from the stressful events that are inevitable in all our life stories and that give rise to our ruminative narratives.

When I next check in with Paola, she tells me that she's been practicing the Body-State Breaker Sigh, Rapid Rescue Muscle Relaxing, and the Rosenberg Technique. She uses the Body-State Breaker Sigh right before she sees or talks to any of her siblings, to help her stay calm during those interactions. She uses Rapid Rescue Muscle Relaxing mainly in response to Will. "Whenever he's joking around and making me the butt of his sophomoric humor, I start squeezing my muscles and releasing them, letting my breath whoosh out. It helps me to release that hot, stinging wind that's blowing into me before it blows me right over." Recently, she did this right in front of Will, after he'd been a jerk about something. He was so startled that he asked her if she was okay. "And my frustration just came erupting out. I told him, 'I'm doing this because I'm so pissed off at you right now. Do *not* talk to me that way—I'm tired of it! It is not okay!'" The big surprise? Will apologized, albeit with a stunned look on his face. "I will take that as progress," Paola tells me. Finally, she uses the Rosenberg Technique every night when she goes to bed. "I yawn myself into my dreams. It's fantastically effective. I'm out in five minutes."

As you experiment with these body-state breakers and find the ones that resonate most with you, remember: Simply tuning in to your sensations tells your nervous system that you matter—pain and all. This tender attention is a quiet but powerful message of safety, one your body may have been craving for a very long time.

NINE

Neuroscience-Based Journaling Techniques

RECENTLY, I HEARD actors Christopher Walken and Ben Stiller talking about their hit television series *Severance* on Stiller's podcast. The two were delving into the idea of being able to step back and separate ourselves from our pain, which is the underlying theme explored in the show.

"Oh, sure," says Walken, who plays a recurrent character. His character has opted to undergo a brain procedure that will "sever" him from emotional pain as soon as he leaves home and steps into the elevator at Lumon, the company where he works. Lumon invented this "severance" procedure, which provides its workers with a daily hit of amnesia about what goes on in their home lives.

"If we could just move past things sometimes," Walken says. "The stuff we carry around. Stuff that [happened] to us when we were kids, that got in our way, the stuff that we carry. It would be nice to have that ability to just throw it out the window and move on."

Wouldn't it be nice. But in a way, this *is* the work we are doing here in this book. Only our work is not about throwing our pain out the window and forgetting it. Rather, the techniques I've been discussing are designed to help you examine the hurt you carry, but to do so from enough of a distance that it's possible for you to get to know it and then make peace with it. Once you do this, your understanding of your own story becomes the doorway to freedom.

Moving your thoughts out of your ruminating mind and onto paper is another practice that helps you to pull back the curtain, step away from these inner machinations, and engage in self-revelation. This is especially true when you write by hand. According to one 2024 study, handwriting leads to widespread brain connectivity and deepens self-insight. Researchers found that when we write out our thoughts by hand, versus typing, we deepen connectivity between the parts of the default mode network involved in self-introspection and embodied sensation, while increasing its communication with other key regions of the brain that help us to reflect on our experience. Typing on digital devices does not offer us this benefit. In a similar study, researchers found that when we read on paper, versus our screens, we process what we're reading more deeply. Taken together, writing on paper, then reading over what we've written, can help free our brains from distressing thoughts while enhancing our brains' ability to intuit, perceive, discern, and decide.

James Pennebaker, professor of psychology at the University of Texas at Austin, is considered the scientific father of the technique known as *writing to heal*, in which you describe stressful experiences in a journal. He intuited some of this decades before neuroscientists peered into the mind to back up this concept with brain scans—and long before he began to study psychology. It was as a young adult that Pennebaker, who suffered from asthma growing up, noticed that his asthma symptoms got worse when he went home to visit his parents for Christmas in West Texas. He had always assumed his asthma was due to the dust that blew into West Texas from New Mexico. But then Pennebaker noticed that whenever his parents came to visit him in Florida, where he lived, he also got asthma attacks. He wondered if unprocessed stress about being in the presence of his parents, and the emotional strain he felt when with them, had somehow impacted his nervous system and physical well-being. His curiosity about how unresolved feelings around family could manifest as physical symptoms eventually led him to develop a psychological-based expressive writing strategy to help individuals process their difficult life experiences.

In studies using college students, Pennebaker asked them to undertake the following steps, and then employ this journaling strategy for fifteen to twenty minutes a day, for four days in a row, or for fifteen to twenty minutes one day a week, for four weeks:

- Write about something distressing that happened in the past that you've been ruminating about and can't stop thinking about. This could be one of the most miserable, frustrating, or difficult life events you've experienced, or any life experience that ignited deep emotions.
- When describing this difficult experience from the past, focus on the facts as best you can recall them, the emotions you felt at the time, *and* any links you see between that negative experience and how it is still affecting you in your life now.
- As you write, don't lift your pencil from the page. Just keep your hand moving as if on automatic pilot, letting your mind and hand do the work for you. Allow the words to fall onto the page as if you're taking dictation from your mind.
- Finally, reflect on the possible benefits of the experience, no matter how unpleasant it was at the time, and write about these benefits. For example, think about how well you coped with the upsetting event and how that resulted in something good, or, if it didn't, how it left you feeling proud of yourself for having done your best. Perhaps this experience made you more aware of personal strengths you didn't know you had until then, or you learned something important about your life goals and values.

Pennebaker found in this and other studies that this two-step journaling strategy of (a) writing about your most difficult experiences on the page and (b) recalling what you've gained as a result of these events helped individuals shift out of "maladaptive rumination," reframe their experience, and switch into "positive coping" in fifteen to twenty minutes. And this wasn't just a mental win. Individuals who wrote about their ruminating thoughts for twenty minutes a day over four days showed improvements in their working memory and mental cognition. They also showed improvements in their bodies' capacity to fight infection. This shift in immune function was profound: Production of mature white blood cells (these are the types of white blood cells produced in our bone marrow and thymus, which help us to stave off and clear infections) increased. They also required fewer doctors' visits compared to those who didn't employ this journaling technique. And in one follow-up study, researchers even showed that writing to heal helped ameliorate the symptoms of asthma. It seems Pennebaker's theory that emotional triggers had worsened his own asthma had been right all along.

Highly expressive individuals (whom Pennebaker called *high disclosers*) who allowed themselves to enter a state of high emotional intensity, letting their fear, anger, or frustration flow onto the page, showed even more improvement in immune function.

As a writer who finds the act of writing a soothing, secure haven from my ruminations, I've long been fascinated by Pennebaker's work. I first started writing in a journal the day after my father's sudden death. I picked up a pink leather diary my parents had given me the previous Christmas, which I'd tucked away in a drawer but had yet to use. I think, as I look back at those entries now, I was writing to my father, as if he might hear me and be swayed by my words to return. I have continued journaling to this day about things that upset or pain me.

But something quite specific to my medical history has always intrigued me about Pennebaker's work. One of the autoimmune conditions that has dogged me across my life is an anomaly—or set of anomalies—in my bone marrow. So Pennebaker's findings, that writing to heal could help with the production of immune cells in one's bone marrow, makes me feel hopeful that when I journal, I'm doing something good for my autoimmune problems. Researchers have since added to Pennebaker's body of research. Duke researchers found that utilizing a six-week expressive writing program among patients decreased their levels of worry and rumination, depression, and stress, and enhanced their resilience. This proved particularly true for individuals who had experienced a recent trauma or significant emotional upheaval—they were able to bring that trauma up and out of the body by getting it onto the page. Other researchers found in a 2020 study that a four-week writing-to-heal program reduced symptoms of depression and stress reactivity.

We all carry invisible scars. We've all had some source of major stress in our lives, and most of us have had traumatic experiences. For some, that adversity is a single seismic event; for others, it's a slow, relentless erosion. In one of the workshops I lead—a ninety-minute writing program I developed specifically to help individuals recovering from adversity—I see this truth again and again in the way a hand scribbles furiously across a page, in the way a tear slips unobtrusively down a cheek. We begin with deceptively simple exercises. I ask participants to respond to prompts—questions I've honed over my three decades as a journalist. These include queries such as: "If you were to give the story of your childhood a movie title, what would it be?"

From here, we move to increasingly deeper questions, such as "What was the hardest year of your childhood?" "When did you feel unseen, unheard, or unimportant?" "What did you long for from your parents but never received?" These questions serve as keys, unlocking the understory of each person's life. I intersperse these and other writing prompts with other tools, including the exercise of drawing the floor plan of your childhood home (which you learned in chapter 6).

After tenderly touching into that understory—your origin

story—we move on to noticing how your past is an active participant in your present, emitting signal flares that ignite deep emotions—and rumination—when new circumstances echo old wounds. After seeing these connections, each person eventually arrives at their own personal code for rumination. It's a moment of recognition: "This is what I keep coming back to." But recognition is only the beginning. From here, we dive into neuroscience-based skills—techniques designed not just to quiet your old stories but to rewrite them so that you can craft a new narrative. One that is powerful, resonant, and true—free at last from the old scripts that have held you back for so long.

After doing this workshop with groups for a decade, I've come to believe that writing to heal is so effective because it requires you to engage in the present moment (hands, eyes, and brain stay engaged in the now as you write words on the page), even as your brain chooses words that call up feelings about events from your past. And you create new meaning out of these experiences, which benefits you long into the future (while also creating a document you can revisit if you want to look back on an earlier you). In this way, you are bridging back and forth across the continuum of your life, and growing wiser, more insightful, more self-compassionate as you do. The truth you already hold inside you, it always turns out, is the most powerful tool you have for transforming you.

The writer Zora Neale Hurston once wrote, "There is no agony like bearing an untold story inside you." It's because journaling gets that story out that it gives us such relief from our agony.

After a recent writing-to-heal workshop, someone told me, "I had an amazing epiphany. That was like a dozen therapy sessions in ninety minutes." I'm not sharing this to push my version of writing to heal; there are, as you've seen, many phenomenal writing-to-heal programs, and Pennebaker's remains the gold standard. The point is that writing can help us rethink our toughest stories, making sense of pain and turning it into progress—often faster than we might expect. I believe this is because writing to heal gives us such direct access to the stories housed in our default mode network—and access to rewriting them in ways that better serve us.

In a 2020 study, psychologists expanded Pennebaker's paradigm to add one step, which is specifically designed to help wrest the brain out of rumination and spiral up into a more positive view of life. They asked participants to add, at the end of the writing protocol:

- Recall the best life events or the happiest times you experienced. Choose one or a couple of them and imagine as if you are in that time. Focus on your feelings, ideas, and emotions and write them down.

Researchers found that adding this flourish was effective at maximizing the results of the Pennebaker technique. Participants reported that "enjoying happiness was a new and somewhat difficult thinking style to learn because they had habitually thought about the negative aspects" of their lives and "rarely thought about" the positive aspects. Freeing participants from their ruminations and engaging them in this new thinking style also improved their working memory. (One note: In this particular study, participants also discussed their writings with a counselor, who helped them pay attention to psychological issues and patterns that arose and redirected them to continue to focus on the positive aspects of their experiences. You, too, might choose to engage in writing-to-heal practices with the support of a counselor or therapist, especially if you feel you need extra guidance and support. It can only deepen your self-awareness and healing.)

Writing to Heal in Action

Sam is finding that journaling to heal is his favorite strategy. Like all of us, he doesn't just ruminate about one thing. In addition to worries about his future in med school, he spends "so much time worrying about the dating scene." When he's on a date, he worries about "whether that girl likes me, and if she doesn't seem to be interested in me, I start down that road of 'What am I doing wrong? What should I do differently? Am I saying the right things, making the right gestures?' I'm not in my own skin." After a date, he can't stop himself from "trying to suss out what she's thinking about me. I second-guess every text, every word I type, when to reach out. And if a girl never responds, I start to think, *Why would she want to date me? Why would anybody?*"

When he's filled with "date doubt," it helps Sam to practice MIST. Recently, after he'd said what he worried was "the wrong thing" while out on a second date with a fellow medical student he "had a crush on," he used this technique to clear the fog of his ruminations. As he did, something new emerged. Old memories came to mind that he hadn't thought about in a long time—experiences of being made fun of by boys at his school when he was in middle and high school. This pattern of rumination felt self-excoriating: *"Here are those familiar video clips about how they don't like me, nobody likes me, which triggers instant self-loathing, like drinking a poison that immobilizes my whole body and makes me want to disappear."*

But Sam needed more than MIST to dive into and release this old storyline. And when he tried Pennebaker's fifteen-minute journaling technique, he found that it helped him to exit that storyline and flip it. He started to appreciate all that he'd gained from having navigated his way through those past experiences, difficult as they were. Not having many friends when he was growing up had led him to channel most of his energy into academics, which had eventually led to his life now: studying at a top medical school. It was a dream he'd always had. His wounds were what had made him want to help others heal. Journaling in this way, which he has made a habit, "shortened the half-life" of his recursive thoughts.

His expanding awareness has resulted in a much more positive outlook on the dating scene. Journaling about all the apprehension and negativity he felt about dating helped him realize that "I'm always coming down hard on myself, which didn't just kill my compassion for myself, it restricted my ability to open up to someone I'm dating, or even to see her beyond the fog of my constant worrying about what to say and what she thinks of me. Without that getting in the way of my being able to listen and respond, I can enjoy getting to know someone, to notice something fascinating, even sacred, about them. That feels new."

The result: The next time he went out on a date with the young woman he was interested in, the interest became mutual, and one date led to more dates and what might be a new relationship. Sam doesn't know where this might lead, but he is sure of one thing: "She probably wouldn't have enjoyed being with me if, every time we were together, I let my negative stories about myself destroy my enjoyment of being with *her*."

Is Sam right? Does ruminating less and being more present make the person he's on a date with more interested in him? I'm pretty sure the answer would be yes—even if we don't have a scientific study to prove it.

Journaling has given Sam some other aha moments—including one that led to a life-changing realization, one in which he was able to "dial into what I really want, what path feels right to me in medicine. When I think back to the moments in which I felt most engaged with my patients, most purposeful, it was during my rotation in child and adolescent psychiatry. The idea of being able to help children and their families—that feels right." Sam has a new adviser in the psychiatry department. When he first told her of his decision, she gave him a hug and told him, "I've seen how engaged children are when you're in the room. We're glad to have you, Sam."

"I never really wanted to be—and I'm not constitutionally suited to be—a surgeon," Sam tells me. "I care more about people's stories and feelings than I do about getting inside of their organs. I guess some part of me hopes if I can help patients see how their experiences shape them, I can create an upstream effect, in which they are healthier moving forward, mentally and physically. I want to offer my skills to help patients with the psychological aspects that influence their healing paradigm, not wait until they come in with a medical emergency and we have to wheel them into the OR and cut them open. There are other ways to open people up, too."

I find this especially brave, since, he confides, "it will mean taking out more money in loans, which I'll have to pay off later. But I'd rather pay off a little more in med school loans to do something that fills me with purpose, than pay back less money for something I never wanted to do in the first place."

The very first time Sam sat with children and their families in a mental health clinic, he knew he'd made the right choice. "I felt that I had finally stepped into the right life. I'm able to connect with the patients sitting in front of me without getting lost in my own self-judging and overanalysis. I'm not intellectualizing. I'm listening, discerning, engaging, offering them the best of me, so I can help them figure out what's best for them." For Sam, digging into the understory of his ruminations has made him "more certain that my take on things is right. I no longer worry so much about whether my read on a situation is right. I know when something feels right." As he speaks these last words, Sam's smile is wider than I've ever seen it—or maybe it's the first time I've seen him smile.

Educational psychologist Kristin Neff, PhD, at the University of Texas at Austin, calls this inner work of being on your own side cultivating your *inner ally.* I like that term because it is precisely this act of becoming an ally to ourselves that helps to rewire our default mode network and free us from the past. In one study of war veterans, the top predictor of *not* having PTSD wasn't how difficult their experiences were but whether they were able, in looking back, to feel compassion for themselves, to bring a warm and caring attitude toward how they met and handled their hardships.

Curiosity about your pain is how you begin to transmute it into a story that's no longer focused on how it can wound you but on how it can heal you. As Suleika Jaouad put it in a recent interview to promote her book *The Book of Alchemy: A Creative Practice for an Inspired Life*, which is all about the practice of journaling: "The goal is not to find an answer. . . . It's to continuously explore and reflect and refine what emerges."

If you love writing as a healing modality, I have one more technique for you. Recently, while on Mel Robbins's podcast, I heard Stanford neurosurgeon and neuroscientist Jim Doty, MD, outline a five-step writing-based practice he teaches. Doty's practice focuses on helping you replace self-doubt and negative thought loops with more empowering thoughts, specifically by "recalibrating" the default mode network. Here's the process:

- Write down a goal you're trying to achieve, or something you're hoping will happen, as if it has already happened. If you're an artist like Virginia, for instance, and you recently submitted your painting to a juried gallery show, it might be, "My work is accepted by X gallery and is in their show."
- Read it silently.
- Read it aloud to yourself.
- Take a moment to really visualize this happening, in as much detail as you can. Using the example of Virginia again, she might imagine the gallery opening, seeing her painting hanging on the wall, feeling the thrill of that accomplishment, imagining who is there with her, catching the scent of cheese and shrimp hors d'oeuvres as they are passed around on trays, hearing the voices of people admiring her painting as they take in the show.
- Repeat it over and over and over.

This, Doty argues, is not just woo-woo positive thinking; it's self-directed neuroplasticity. Simple writing practices like these can help you embrace small, steady changes that invite you to express yourself—your aliveness, your "mattering"—more fully.

For those of us who journal regularly, it's a process so powerful and healing that we can feel, as Suleika Jaouad has said, that it's a lifesaver. Jaouad has had three bouts of cancer over the last fifteen years, the latest one having been diagnosed in August of 2024. She's journaled for as long as she can remember, but the practice became even more urgent for her once she received her first diagnosis of cancer. And it has remained so. "I don't know how I would have managed knowing that I'll never be cured if I didn't have this sacred container where I get to be my most unedited, unvarnished self."

TEN

Let the Positive Do Battle with the Negative—and Win!

EVEN ONCE WE use MIST to see and recognize our personal rumination codes, practice ballistic interrupters, employ body-state breakers, and journal to heal, we still need a next layer of strategies to help us enter, and remain in, a more positive emotional state. The absence of positive emotions is as big a risk factor to your mental and physical well-being as how frequently you ruminate. So how can you generate positive emotions in those moments when you are feeling overwhelmed by runaway negative thoughts?

One of the most empowering ways to accomplish this is to learn how to introduce positive imagery into the same mental space as your negative thoughts and allow the positive to win out over the negative. Surprising as this sounds, there are actually some fast, actionable, neuroscience-based hacks that can help you cultivate the opposite feelings from those your ruminations give rise to, visualizing and embodying those positive emotions and thoughts so vividly that it's as though they are real and you're feeling them now. This will allow them to fully register deep inside your brain and your body, all the way down to your mitochondria. On a neurobiological level, you're creating neuroplasticity through a process known as *neuromodulation;* you're changing how your synapses fire in ways that support clarity, intuition, ingenuity, proactive thinking, and purposeful, choice-driven action. This, in turn, promotes more feel-good chemicals in your brain, including dopamine, oxytocin, and serotonin. On a felt level, you will enjoy moving through the world in a more expansive, creative, and aware state.

Most of these techniques use positive mental imagery. Visualization is a remarkably powerful way to keep us out of the negative thought patterns that cause us to spiral down into mind drama. In a 2023 study, psychologists at Oregon State University showed that *visualizing* positive mental imagery is a considerably more effective way to exit rumination and regulate our nervous systems than *verbalizing* positive thoughts. This makes sense: Creating mental imagery is a much more immersive brain endeavor than putting thoughts into words, because it requires a coordinated effort across your entire connectome—the map of neural connections linking various regions of the brain. Moreover, imagining positive mental pictures and events lights up the same parts of the brain that become engaged when we see and experience those things in real life. Every time you take a few minutes to embody these practices, you're leveraging the remarkable power of your brain to upgrade the narrative of who you believe you are and who you know you are capable of becoming.

There are a multitude of techniques that can help you to create that positive imagery in your brain. Below are a few of the strategies that I've found particularly useful. You can try them all out or just zero in on one that seems to speak to you. Whatever you choose, include it in the collection of tools you use to help you shift and stay out of rumination.

Two-Roads Visualization

Paola has realized, through excavating her ruminations and their origin stories, that she needs more help to heal if she is to feel whole. In an act of great bravery, she's started seeing a therapist for the first time in her life. Her therapist has taught her the following technique, she tells me. It's based on the concept of *psychological flexibility*—the ability to hold two conflicting ideas in mind to see more clearly how we feel and the choices that we need to make.

Paola is particularly drawn to this concept because she feels she's at a "fork in the road" in her marriage. She wants a future with Will, and she believes that can happen. But she wants the future to be one in which they both grow and change. Otherwise, she feels, she may have to take her own path. Part of the work her therapist has given her is to be able to visualize the possibility of what a future with Will might look like. And this requires Paola to cultivate feelings that are the opposite of those dredged up by the litany of resentful judgments she's written down in her "Will Book." "I've spent so much time caught up in rumination about the ways he's let me down that my muscles for emotional intimacy, and how to foster that, have become atrophied," she tells me. "How can I know if we can build a better marriage if I don't have the skills for closeness and connection myself?"

The technique her therapist has taught her—the Two-Roads Visualization—is helping Paola to do that. It takes five minutes—and, for those of you who enjoy video games, it's a little bit like playing a video game in your head. But in this visualization, you generate your own mental imagery, both positive and negative. Here's how to practice it:

First, visualize two roads in your mind, and imagine yourself standing where those two roads diverge. (Yes, this calls to mind Robert Frost's poem "The Road Not Taken.") Here, you have a choice about which road to take. If you follow the long, dark road to your left, you'll encounter and inhabit all your gloomy, unpleasant thoughts, imagery, and stories—a land you don't want to dwell in. There, it's sleeting and the weather is abysmal. If you were to travel that road, you would marinate in all the past resentments, emotions, and stories that ignite your ruminations. You can just imagine the dire sights you would see as well as the cacophony of unpleasant, discordant sounds you would hear on that well-trodden, misery-making terrain.

Alternately, you can choose to start down the road to your right—a better road. To fully orient yourself onto the right-hand path and give it a tangible, physical reality, you must literally turn your body to the right. (Yes, literally. Whether you're sitting or standing, turn your body so that you're facing to your right. If you're lying down, roll toward your right. Making this physical shift matters; it signals your default mode network to reorient itself.) Now, imagine yourself walking down that tree-lined and flower-strewn road on a beautiful day as you encounter people and places you treasure.

Continue to imagine yourself walking down the road to the right and let your imagination take over. On this road, you will relive meaningful moments, see people (including those who are now gone) who truly loved you, revisit places you love, while also enjoying experiences that are new and exciting. What those future experiences will be depends on what you hope they will be. Picture them in your mind. As you move forward on the road, bring scenes alive as if you are populating them in a video game. Visualize the grass growing and the trees bursting into full bloom, smell the lavender in the fields. Gently stroke the faces of people you love, or have loved, as you encounter them along this path. The goal here is to self-create a world containing all the most heartfelt moments you've ever experienced and hope yet to experience, bringing it all alive so that you can see, hear, feel, taste, and smell it as vividly as you can. Who is there? What are their voices saying? What does the air smell like? What sounds do you hear?

If you get distracted and find your mind returning to the left-hand path, know that that's perfectly normal. Simply reroute yourself by turning your body back toward the "right" path. Continue to populate it with loved ones, treasured places, beautiful memories, aspirations, and possibilities. As you do this, connect with the feelings and emotions you'd like to lean into as you relive them or imagine them happening in the future.

This practice is powerful for two reasons. First, studies show that each time we rejuvenate past joyful experiences in our minds, we reinforce neural pathways that will help us to recall our life's highlights long into our future. Second, this visualization helps us to see our future selves as real. We often treat our future selves as if they are strangers; we can't concretize the idea of who we will be in a year, or two, or twenty, and this makes it harder for us to do the things we need to do today to make a better future. Someone can tell you when you're twenty to lift weights so you don't get osteoporosis when you're sixty, but since you can't see that future self as a real person, it's hard to feel the motivation to lift weights.

The more you practice the Two-Roads Visualization, the easier it will be for your mind to instantly recall the most meaningful moments of your life, while building a path toward a better future, in whatever way you need to, instead of meandering down the old, dark alley of your mind drama.

What does this look like for Paola? When Paola imagines heading down the road to the left, she starts to feel "re-consumed and digested by those old storylines. That's the road that is always calling me. I see creepy trees with long limbs stretching out to ensnare me. I hear the old shitty voices calling out belittling things—from my siblings, especially. But from Will, too. And I start flipping through my 'Will Book' to remember all the mean, stupid things he's said to me. Then I think, *There they all are, collaborating in this caricature of an idea of who I am, this name-calling,* and suddenly I think: *Why should I collaborate in it, too, by replaying it all? What if I walk down a different road? What will I find there?*"

Paola then turns her body to the right and walks down that road instead. "I try to create this beautiful landscape as I go, populating it with all the best moments I've had with Will, but also all the best moments I've had in my life when I was alone in nature, or hiking somewhere, or staring at something beautiful, or in a new city by myself, and I felt, *Wow, I'm pretty good company,* and enjoyed that solitude, that sense of solo adventure." From here, she begins populating it with more moments like these—with Will, and also by herself—which stem from her imagination. They may not have happened yet, but they feel real. And they feel—"happy."

As Paola continues down this road, so many moments "start to come back to me of times when Will has been kind, when he has shown up for me and let me know how much he cares. Once on an aid trip, our tire blew out on the road, and we were going to have to spend hours dealing with getting it fixed since we'd forgotten to bring a spare. Looking at me, Will knew how exhausted I was, and he asked our colleagues, who were in another jeep, to take me back to our offices while he took care of getting our jeep fixed. Or how every morning he makes a huge pot of oatmeal with nuts and berries and gives half of it to me."

Once Paola gets her brain humming in this more integrated way, by cultivating the opposite feelings from those that populate her usual ruminative downward spiral, she begins to disprove her reflexive assumptions that her husband is irredeemably immature or incapable of being caring. She starts to notice more moments when Will does show love, concern, and respect. Here, Paola is activating her brain's filtering system; by shining a spotlight on these moments, she sees more of them. And this leads to "other possibilities." By which Paola means, "Maybe this impasse I'm seeing between us isn't this big, catastrophic problem I'm telling myself it is. Maybe I can redirect some of the brainpower I've been donating to my mind drama to do something more constructive: sit down and talk to Will about my fears. And then I think, *Well, what are my fears?* And it turns out my fear is pretty simple: As I get older, what if my body and stamina change and I can't or don't want to do all the adventurous high-risk things he still wants to do? Or what if I need his help because I'm ill? What will happen as he gets older? We can't just avoid the topic; we will both get old one day.

"Yesterday, I mentioned to Will that my back hurt, and he said, 'Omigod, you're turning into a hypochondriac! You sound just like my grandma!' Instead of getting flooded with memories of all his other dismissive comments and withdrawing into myself, I calmly reminded him of the various health problems I'd been diagnosed with recently and asked him to stop using them against me. He was quiet, and then he said, 'Fair point. Fair point.' Then I asked him, 'Are *you* afraid of getting older, of *your* body having failings and vulnerabilities?' He said, 'Hell yes, that's my worst nightmare.' I said, 'Maybe we need to figure out a plan for what will happen if one of us is ill.' That led us into a deeper discussion, and we left the conversation agreeing to set up an appointment with a financial adviser." By not reacting to his comments or going down those "darker, twistier mental roads, I'm able to learn what's driving not just my fears but his." And suddenly the future, the what-ifs, don't seem so overwhelming for Paola.

She has, she tells me, developed a shorthand method to quickly channel her newfound constructive mental framework in just a few seconds, based on her work with the Two-Roads Visualization. "If I'm getting sucked into reliving a litany of past grievances, replaying things Will has said to me, I do a quick emergency intervention before my brain gets totally hijacked." First, she uses a ballistic interrupter: "We're not going there! Because it leads nowhere, and I'd rather move forward." Then, invoking the two roads, "I glance to my right as if I'm looking at something out of the corner of my eye, and that instantly helps me to conjure up my right-hand road. I can do this at the grocery store, and no one knows I'm doing it. It helps me leave behind all my fear-based thoughts from the past so I can focus on what is true and not true, and what might be possible in the future, without all that noise in my head."

As a result of this work, Paola has learned that "the degree to which I'm caught up in obsessive thought spirals is usually in direct proportion to the degree that I'm not feeling my feelings. Or I'm not attuned to how constricted my body has become. Or I'm not listening to what I need for me." Each time Paola gets caught up in "judging Will, I try to stop in the middle of it and ask myself, 'What am I trying not to feel right now?' Once I allow myself to accept and honor all my emotions, I can let go of the story, and the judgment evaporates."

The Flash Technique

If you were to list the strategies you think would be most effective at defusing your emotions after a stressful conversation or a disturbing event, you'd probably assume you'd need to recall, replay, and unpack the who, what, when, and where to understand why you felt so intensely about it. But the Flash Technique is built on a premise that is the opposite of this idea.

According to psychotherapist Tom Zimmerman, who trains therapists in this methodology, it offers us a unique way to process challenging life experiences. "We're often drawn to ruminate about and replay what happened to us, hoping for a solution or a catharsis, but nothing changes. With the Flash Technique, we're working with memory in a nonintuitive way. You get into what happened to you without having to actually get *into* it."

What I find intriguing and hopeful about the Flash Technique is that it allows us to bypass our default mode network's proclivity to ruminate and instead switch, remarkably quickly, into healthy emotional processing, which happens below the level of our conscious awareness. Zimmerman explains, "We're allowing ourselves to bring past difficult experiences into the present in a way that teaches our nervous system we're safe. We do this by showing our nervous system that these experiences are *not* still happening to us here and now. When we let our nervous systems know that they're over, they're in the past, and something more positive is happening now, they won't be a source of rumination anymore."

Zimmerman has volunteered to meet over Zoom and walk

me through the practice, which was first developed by clinical psychologist Philip Manfield, PhD, as an adjunct to his EMDR work with patients. EMDR, or Eye Movement Desensitization and Reprocessing, is a psychotherapy treatment that helps people process traumatic memories by having them focus on the trauma, while engaging in bilateral stimulation (such as side-to-side eye movements). The Flash Technique, on the other hand, helps to reduce the intensity of lingering wounds without dwelling on the painful details; instead, after identifying the trauma, you quickly shift your focus to a positive thought. The Flash Technique also differs in its use of eye movement, employing the simple act of blinking rather than the bilateral stimulation used in EMDR.

This practice requires about fifteen minutes. You'll want to prepare in the following ways:

Gather Your "Resources." Your resources are both mental and physical. The mental resources include coming up with a calm scene that you can focus on as you do this exercise. Your calm scene can be anything that, for you, brings up a sense of calm and relaxation. You might imagine or remember a scene such as a beautiful hike in the woods, dinner with someone you love and with whom you've always felt safe (whether that person is alive or not), or even just the sight of your cats curled up around each other in sleep. "Bring to mind anything you love—your baby's big cheeks, golden retrievers chasing tennis balls," Zimmerman advises. If you can't think of a positive memory or scene to work with, or you're just not feeling very imaginative, it's perfectly fine to pull up a YouTube video that makes you feel relaxed and calm. "Maybe you like watching videos of scuba divers on the Great Barrier Reef, or of people baking or painting. Whatever it is, if it fills you with calm, this will be your calm scene to which you will repeatedly return." Then you also have to come up with a target memory—of something upsetting enough that it still has the power to send you into rumination—that you want to be able to move past.

Your physical resources are what you will use to ground yourself. Maybe you want to sit in a favorite chair, light a scented candle, or put a vase of flowers or a photo of someone you love nearby so you'll have something beautiful to look at. Whatever adds to your sense of being present and safe will help you to ground.

Zimmerman asks me to identify a calm scene for myself, and because it is soon after the holidays, I choose the first thing that comes to mind: my husband and son and daughter and me sitting in front of the fire together on Christmas morning a few weeks earlier, opening gifts under the twinkling lights of the Christmas tree. It had been a challenging year. My son had recently had surgery, I'd been managing a more serious autoimmune flare than I'd had in some years, my mother-in-law was in hospice, my mother had become nearly blind and needed more help, and . . . well, you know. Life was doing what life does. That Christmas, everyone had been a little extra thoughtful, giving gifts to one another that showed they'd paid attention to what people had mentioned months earlier about what they needed or wished they had. Replacing all the toxic black plastic utensils in the kitchen with wooden ones because someone had read an article and said what a good idea that would be. The coat someone had mentioned loving that previous spring, which had later gone on sale, was a surprise hit and fit perfectly. The poetry book someone had said in passing they'd always wished they'd read in high school. A one-year pass to a favorite botanical garden. But it wasn't about the gifts in the stockings and beneath the tree. Of course it wasn't. It was about being together, so happy to be together, and nowhere else. Family as a hard-won haven from the storm of life.

"Do you have it?" Zimmerman asks.

"I do," I said, the smile already on my face as I immersed myself in my neurally soothing mental slideshow—seeing the dogs in front of the fire, hearing the sounds of the fire crackling, of paper being ripped off all the carefully wrapped presents, smelling the lingering aromas of the tea, coffee, hot chocolate, and maple syrup–covered waffles we'd just had for breakfast, soon to be replaced by the scent of a standing rib roast and oven-roasted potatoes. As for grounding myself, I had a mug of my favorite cup of tea, and my dog Winnie was curled up at my feet, should I need help staying in the present.

Identify Your Target Memory. Zimmerman advises starting small with "the little fish," or memories and scenarios that are not overwhelming. Find something that's generating recurrent blips of worry, brooding, rumination, sadness—those difficult moments and losses you're having trouble letting go of—but avoid anything that's too traumatic. "Later, if you want to, you can work your way up to the bigger fish," Zimmerman adds. (One note: While this version of the Flash Technique can be a self-guided practice, if you follow along with a practitioner such as Manfield or Zimmerman on YouTube, it's important to work directly with a practitioner to process more traumatic memories.)

"Do you have something?" he asks me.

"Is it okay if it is something I've been working to process for years?"

"That's fine, as long as it's not bringing up feelings that are completely overwhelming right now," Zimmerman says.

Somehow, in conjuring up Christmas morning, I had begun to think about Christmas mornings as a child, and the twelve I'd enjoyed with my father before he died. My father had had a saying, "Let's go make a memory!" before any fun family event or gathering, and Christmas morning was no exception—he went big. In all the years since he died, especially once I had a family of my own, I've tried to carry on that tradition, while also wishing so much that he could be here to join in. Often, no matter how joyous they are, family gatherings have a big hole in them—a father-size hole.

Like all children who have lost a parent early in life, I wanted him to see what I've made of my life, and to meet my husband and my children. I've always hoped he would be proud to know that I became a writer, just like him. And because he was the one person in my life who "saw" me, the one who made me feel I mattered, I knew he would "see" what I see in the people I love. It would have tickled him to see how his grandson chases hard, ethical questions, just as he did, how he goes out of his way to show up for other people, and how much he possesses of my dad's irrepressible, quick wit. My son is so much like my father that the fact that they have never met has always pained me. He would have smiled, too, to see how my daughter possesses his uncanny perceptiveness about other people, and to know that she, like his mother, is a born poet. And I like to imagine how well he and my husband would have gotten along. Like my father, my husband, in his own way, has devoted his life to public service and the public good.

Much as I have moments of missing my father in the midst of happy times, it's in life's harder moments that I feel his absence most keenly: his calm steering of the ship in the storm; the feeling, in his presence, that I was never alone; his way of offering up just the right words at the right moment.

During my son's recent surgery, I'd had a particularly intense bout of longing for my father and his guidance. My son's surgery took place in the same hospital where my father died. As I sat in the family waiting room, expecting the surgeon to come out at any minute and give me a progress report, I began to grow agitated. The surgery was taking far longer than anticipated—he'd already been in the OR for an hour longer than we'd been told to expect. My husband had gone home to feed and walk the dog and hadn't returned yet. A few chairs away, a father and daughter were waiting together, clutching hands, her head resting on his shoulder, as they waited for their loved one to come out of surgery. I had to swallow hard not to burst into tears or panic or some combination of the two. I began to pace the waiting room.

My son was in for a minor surgery. (Later, we would find out all had gone swimmingly, but given my son's history—he'd had major abdominal surgery as a newborn—the surgeon had done exploratory surgery first; she was being careful and safe.) But I didn't know the cause of the delay at the time. Fear became embarrassment, shame, at how worked up I was becoming. Why was I getting so . . . hysterical? He would be fine! I was here to support my son. How would I soothe him when he came out of the operating room if I was flooded by my own emotions? I didn't want to put that on him, be that kind of mom who needs someone to take care of her when she is the one who should be doing the caretaking.

Zimmerman must see by the tears pricking my eyes that I have a target memory. "You have one?"

"Yes." I nod, confident I've finally landed on a memory that will work in this context.

"Good. But don't replay it all. If it's replaying right now like a movie in your head, stop the reel, know that it's there, and set it aside. Now we're going to take that memory and put it away in a container."

I gulp. "Okay, yes." I stop the scene replaying in my head as best I can.

Your Container. This one is simple. Imagine a container that you can put your target memory away in.

"Once you think of that container, you're going to put your target memory in it and send it far, far away from you to the other side of Pluto," Zimmerman says. "Any container will do."

In my mind, I visualize putting my target memory inside an army transport plane, the type with huge rear cargo doors that slam definitively shut. I describe it to Zimmerman.

"Okay, great. Put your target memory in there, watch the doors close, and send that plane far, far away," he coaches.

I play this hospital waiting room scene out in my mind, and as I send my memory off in the cargo plane, I gesture, throwing my arm up and over my head as if I'm slinging something into space, to the other side of the known world.

"Good! I like that gesture you're making with your arm! Like you're really sending that target memory far, far away."

Your Vacuum. "You want to imagine you have a vacuum within reach—you'll see why as we go on," Zimmerman explains.

Now that Zimmerman has helped me identify my grounding resources, my calm scene, and my target memory, we are ready to begin bringing pieces of that target memory into working memory for processing. To do this, he'll be using the *blink technique.*

"Bring up your calm scene," he instructs me. As I do, I re-inhabit it, the four of us on Christmas morning, healthy, here, together, the twinkling lights, the fire, the dogs, the smiles, the tea and chocolate, the rip of paper, the laughter, the deep, shared connection we have built, worked for, and treasure.

I'm deep in this happy dream when Zimmerman says, "Blink!"

I blink rapidly six or seven times.

"Okay, reenter your calm scene."

I do, and a few minutes later, he says it again: "Blink!"

We go through this six times—I immerse myself in my calm scene, he interrupts it to tell me to blink, I do, and then I return to . . . well . . . Christmas morning.

After six rounds of blinking at specific intervals, he asks me to check in with my target memory. "Start the reel with that scene, and as soon as you meet any activation, anything at all that feels charged, stop, and go back to your calm scene."

As the reel unspools, I see myself in the hospital's family waiting room, blinking back tears, that hard gulp in my throat, the old bottomless fear, and the shame around that wound that never seems to heal.

"Okay, good. Bring out your vacuum to vacuum out any residual activation—any sense of dread, shame, guilt, if it's there. Now put it back in the container on the plane and send that target memory up into space. Then return to your calm scene."

Again I go back to Christmas morning. All is well, all are safe, all is love.

We repeat this process for the next fifteen minutes, though it feels to me like five. With each round, my calm scene feels realer and realer, as if I were in it right now. I almost expect to look up and see that it is Christmas morning, still.

Each time we touch on my target memory, I get a little bit further into the scene in which I'm waiting for news during my son's surgery, trying not to lose it, trying not to be that hysterical woman in the waiting room. Each time, this target memory becomes a little less painful. As my sense of calm expands, I can feel something deeper going on. My grief is transmuting into something else. I talk to my father in my head and tell him, "I love you, Dad, I love you. I've missed you and loved you every day. I am letting my child's grief go now; this wound of missing you in all the best moments and the hardest ones. And I want you to know, I am okay. I turned out okay. And I have this beautiful family, you would love them, and they would love you."

Then, something astonishing happens. I return one last time to my calm scene, to Christmas morning in our living room. And my father is there. Sitting on the sofa, in front of the fire, the dogs at his feet. He is there, though no one can see him but me. But *I* saw him, my father, sitting on the sofa, watching, taking it all in, smiling, and I saw—no, felt—the joy he felt in observing that everything really was okay. He'd always known me, known me in my core, essential self, and I had always known him, and in some intangible way I knew he knew my family, too. I saw him, sitting with me during my son's surgery, next to me, holding my hand. And I knew then, as I have sometimes known in other moments of my life, that we had never really said goodbye and never would. He is still with me, as is that sense of safety he had instilled in me.

Afterward, Zimmerman asks me, "How was that?"

I tell him what came up for me.

"Does it leave you thinking about yourself any differently?"

"I don't feel so much pain. I don't feel so much shame about my pain," I say.

"That's when we know that the Flash Technique is working," he says. "Because we end up thinking about ourselves and our experiences differently."

Whenever I feel that old, familiar pain these days, instead of falling into the grief of a loss that lives forever, my mind goes to that bittersweet feeling of connection I experience whenever I think about my father, and about my own small family, whom I know he would have loved. I smile the kind of smile that comes when we tap into the timelessness of love.

This is what can happen when the default mode network is able to process painful memories and charged emotions without our having to consciously attend to the original pain of our memory.

Your Fear Is Your Friend

One way to cultivate the opposite feelings of those generated by rumination and dissolve the ironclad grip your default mode network can have on your life is to actively challenge your negative beliefs and, by doing so, prove them wrong. By pressure testing your consistent, negative thoughts with opposite thoughts, you can help rob your ruminations of their colossal strength. (One caveat here: This technique is useful for stubborn, ruminative thought loops—but if you're facing a crisis, or an abusive or otherwise dangerous situation, more help and support are obviously needed.)

Paola has tried this strategy, which is based on the work of sociologist Martha Beck, PhD, and applied it to her ruminations about her situation with Will. Recently, we met up for coffee. When Paola walked into the café, something subtle but unmistakable had shifted. Her posture told the story before she spoke: shoulders squared, chin lifted, the slight habitual stoop replaced by a quiet confidence. Her gray hair was newly cropped and curling with a kind of liberated ease. But as we talked, I saw the transformation ran deeper.

Over coffee, Paola demonstrates for me a technique of Beck's that is premised on the idea that suffering can be our greatest ally if we let it speak, because it can tell us what we most need to know.

Paola begins this process by asking herself this question: "What is one of my scariest thoughts when I let my greatest fear speak?" What sets off alarm bells in Paola's nervous system is this: "My greatest fear is that I've spent decades with a man who was critical and immature and that was so, so, so stupid of me."

Once you let your fear speak in this way, you can turn that fear-thought around to see something you didn't see before. "Suffering always tells you the opposite of what you need to know," Beck teaches.

I venture to Paola, "So I guess your question would be: What is the opposite of your fear that you did something stupid by marrying Will?"

"That I did something so incredibly smart; I married the person I needed to marry to heal myself." Paola's eyes light up, as if she's surprised by her own thoughts. "If I hadn't married him, I wouldn't be challenged to do this work and learn how to stand up for myself."

"How does that feel?"

"All this relief is racing through my body. It's like I've taken the teeth out of the fear."

"How does that change things moving forward, if at all?"

"It feels like I'm freeing up some kind of kinetic energy to work on our marriage, versus staying in the drama about me, my stupid choices, and the minutiae of our marriage. Instead of my anger and disappointment guiding me, I can let the opposite of that feeling guide me."

What I see in Paola is the visible result of internal work. The self-realization we achieve by decoding our ruminations and working through what our emotions are signposting for us isn't about denying discomfort or past struggles; it's about showing up honestly to our own reality and choosing to grow from it. Paola is no longer shrinking to fit old narratives. She's taller now, not because she's grown but because she's finally standing in her own truth.

Later that afternoon, after getting off the phone with a difficult friend (well, an acquaintance) with whom I've had a stressful conversation, I decide to try this technique for myself. This acquaintance had asked me to do something for her that I didn't feel good about. Every instinct told me not to. It wasn't nefarious—it just didn't meet my gut test for something I felt right about doing. (I'm keeping things deliberately vague here.) She kept texting me, pressing, cajoling. My vague responses were insufficient to the task of shutting down this enormous ask. (Yeah, I don't like confrontation.) Finally, I texted back, "Let's move on from this. I care about you, but I'm not able to help you with this one." After several days, I still hadn't heard back from her. From the minute I'd sent my text, I'd felt that old gut-wrench of doubt. Maybe I was the one who was wrong? Maybe I'd been entirely selfish in being unwilling to extend myself, my time, my resources so far on her behalf? My mind kept racing as my stomach clenched. Geesh, had I been a jerk? No wonder she hadn't texted me back.

I applied Beck's strategy to see how it worked, asking myself, "Am I being shortsighted about this friendship? Did I just do something really stupid?"

Here's what came back to me (yes, it came back to me from my own head): "You felt really taxed by this request and knew it wasn't right, and you just did something wonderful for yourself!" And I realized, in that moment, yes, I *had* done something wonderful for myself. I had detached myself from a situation—and if I was honest, probably a friendship—that had often felt overwhelming and a little bit off.

By allowing myself to be guided by the opposite of my fear, I was able to realize that saying no in this situation wasn't a sign that there is something wrong with me but instead an indication that I know how to make a wise choice. I had made suffering my friend—my adviser of sorts—and sent my nervous system a self-affirming message instead of the old messages about my always doing everything wrong and being "the problem."

What we're going for with all these tools is genuine self-knowledge that allows us to become more reliable narrators of our own stories, so that we are no longer creating dark narratives out of all the difficult and challenging interactions that happen to us. And this, it seems to me, is a meta-skill we all need more of to help us navigate our complex lives.

ELEVEN

The Power of Rest to Free You from Your Overthinking

ALL THIS CHANGE requires effort, I know. Still, I hope that by now you've found that showing up for yourself in these ways feels pleasurable (and is the antithesis of work). I hope you are finding that it feels good to wake up on your own side—perhaps for the first time in your life. Nevertheless, it seems fitting, after all this effort, to pivot and talk about the power of deep rest, and how this simple state can support your efforts to free yourself from your Inner Defeatist.

There is a constant conversation taking place between our brains and the world out there, but we aren't meant to be in thinking mode all the time. The clamor of our media-driven world—what C. S. Lewis once called "the great cataract of nonsense that pours from the press" (and Lewis didn't even live in the era of social media or online news)—deafens us to what matters most while increasing the volume of our overthinking.

Your default mode network needs true quiet—a break from being caught up in the long-standing narratives about your worth, or what others might think of you, that intrude into your thought stream. This requires that you give yourself permission to rest. On a practical level, it means scheduling in periods of silence so that you can take a solid, substantial break from responding to others' needs, chasing worries, or jumping into action as you whack away at your endless to-do list. Many of us were raised with the idea that to slow down, or worse, lie down, is analogous to being lazy, indolent, selfish. Our parents might have given us this idea, a notion that was no doubt pushed on them, for it is part of the great American work ethic. But giving in to the need for extra rest is anything but lazy; research shows it's neuroprotective and makes us more resilient and productive in the long run.

How do you give yourself periods of true rest during your too-busy days? Here are some techniques that can help you to achieve deeper-than-normal rest, while lessening your recursive ruminations.

I hope it goes without saying that whatever road to rest you choose, you will need to silence your phone and darken your screens and set them all aside.

Lie Down—on the Ground

When we lie or sit down in old, familiar places, like our beds or favorite armchairs, our minds are quick to engage in the old, familiar thought patterns of mind drama, because that's what we've done in that same spot so many times before. According to Alan Fogel, professor of psychology at the University of Utah, we can break this pattern by lying on the ground (or floor). This serves as an excellent tool to help us avoid ruminating. In our Western culture, "we don't have a lot of spaces for restoration," he argues. "There are no time-outs. There's no recess." By lying on the ground, or on the floor, we are literally gaining a different perspective. As we feel the hardness or coolness of the floor beneath us, we experience things differently in our bodies. As we gaze up from the floor, we see everything from a new vantage point. This unfamiliarity signals our brains to open up and let go, which allows our thought streams to dissipate. As we acclimate to this different perspective, we are less focused on our thoughts and more likely, Fogel found, "to just be."

If you're able to lie on the ground outside, you might add in another sensory element. Touch grass, or a stone, or the trunk or root of the tree you're lying beneath. This further signals your body and mind to let go, rest, and be. In one study of fifty-four female university students, touching one's hand to grass for just five minutes significantly reduced blood pressure and stress levels compared to touching artificial (plastic) turf.

Sam has, no surprise, been short on rest throughout medical school, and things have only become more hectic of late, now that he's decided to pursue child and adolescent psychiatry. It's a daunting time. "I'm racing toward this new thing that excites me, and I don't have time to stop and recharge. I worry I'm behind everyone else. Seems like the only time I sit down is to work or drive or eat. And a lot of times I eat while I work, or I'm stuffing a sandwich in my mouth as I drive."

"How is that working out for you?" I ask.

"On the one hand, I feel like the future is this exciting puzzle to solve. I know I won't have all the answers, but I want to find them, one case, one patient at a time. But I also notice the more I rush and the less I rest, the more I get caught up in my old thinking: *Will this work out? Am I making a mistake? I'm disappointing a lot of people! What do I know about psychiatry? I'm too messed up myself to help other people! Who am I kidding?*" Sam has a moniker for this: "Stinking thinking."

Part of the reason Sam keeps hitting Replay on his stinking thinking is that those stories are still running in his default mode network, which rarely rests to reboot—because Sam never does.

When Sam was growing up, no one ever gave him permission to take time for himself. "It was seen as a negative. If I wasn't doing homework or just wanted to play or read a book, my dad would say, 'What are you doing? Why are you such a sloth?' The busier I was, the more my parents respected me. My dad used to say, 'You have to push hard if you want to be somebody in this world! Or do you want to be a loser?' "

Sam shares an apartment with friends but has no time to hang out with them. He's usually at the university teaching hospital, where every moment feels competitive and rushed. "A lot of my interactions are not nurturing; they're situations in which I'm being evaluated. They make me second-guess myself and my decisions even more. I've figured out that when I start ruminating, it's a sign that I need to step back from interacting with people and find more quiet, more stillness, in my day. If I get home and one more request from someone, or the sound of my phone dinging with incoming texts makes me feel exhausted or resentful, I know I need to be alone to do a reset, clear my head. If the sound of my roommate chewing makes me want to live by myself, I need to be alone. I need more time to recuperate from all the small interactions and asks and tasks of the day. And by that, I don't mean meditating or going for a walk. I mean alone time without any agenda, without any human interaction, without any goal—I just need to let my mind rest."

Sam is trying to find more opportunities to address this need. His current go-to is to lie down on the ground, touching grass, something he hasn't done since he was a kid. "On my breaks, I go outside the med school building and lie on the grass on the quad and just stare at the sky. I can feel the grass brushing against my skin in the breeze. Everything falls away. Even five minutes is restorative. Yesterday, I watched a flock of starlings swoop and dive in this almost otherworldly choreography. I tucked my fingers into little tufts of grass as I watched the last bit of daylight fall across the trees. Suddenly, I felt as if nothing in the world could ever bother me again. That small reset got me through the next twelve hours with a renewed perspective, and it quashed my stupider thoughts."

An Old-Fashioned "Lie-Down"

When I was growing up, one of my friends' mothers used to have a "lie-down" every afternoon, at four o'clock, rain or shine. She lived well into her nineties and had a clear mind until the day she died. When I became a mother, and several of my friends also had newborns and toddlers, one of my best friends did the same thing. Every day, while her baby slept, she rested on her bed, by herself. (No phone, no digital accoutrements—we didn't have them back then!) She didn't sleep, but that wasn't the point; she was resting, she said, and that made all the difference to the remainder of her day. To be fair, she was working part-time from home and had a part-time babysitter, but rather than get more work done or catch up on laundry when her baby slept, she recuperated. I can't tell you how much I admired that. (Though her son is grown now, she still rests, marinating in stillness, every day—I admire that, too.)

As for me, I never learned from my friend; I used my children's nap times to write and meet deadlines—to my own detriment, as I now see. There was one exception to my inability to rest during the day, which was inspired by a conversation I had the first time I went on a writing residency. As the director was showing me around, I asked her why, even though I had a room and a bed in the building where writers were housed, I also had a bed in my writing studio. Were we expected to be working into the wee hours of the night? "Hardly," she laughed. "We put beds in all the studios because we know that to create, you need to spend a lot of time lolling around doing nothing while your creative thoughts unfurl." And so, because I had been given permission, I did sometimes lie down, especially when I could feel my mind trying to process choices I had to make about structure and word choice. And it helped. I generated better work.

Despite what I learned about its benefits, however, it was many years before I began to carry this practice over to my normal life, and I still find it takes a very concerted mental effort to get myself to stop what I'm doing and lie down for twenty minutes. I wonder if you—like me, like Sam—have felt this, too; that you should only rest when you have absolutely nothing left to give. If so, you're not alone. In one study of eighteen thousand people from 134 countries, researchers found that most of us have a conflicted relationship with rest and associate the very word with feeling guilty. But some of our greatest artists and thinkers seem to have had no such hesitation. Both Albert Einstein and Leonardo da Vinci, for example, carved out time each day for "free-floating periods of thought." Leonardo would often sit thinking in front of a painting for half a day. Einstein liked to drift aimlessly on water in a wooden boat he called the *Tinef* (Yiddish for "piece of junk") while he did some of his thinking.

There was a reason these great minds took this time, according to neuroscientist Nancy Andreasen, MD, PhD. She studied what happens to the brain when we enter a resting state and free our minds to wander and find their own way, and found that during such free-floating thought periods, the brain begins to default to creativity, "gathering information from the senses and from elsewhere in the brain [to] link it all together in potentially novel ways" . . . using the brain's "most human and complex parts." Andreasen's findings underscore the fact that long, recuperative periods of silence are healing for our ruminating minds.

Non-Sleep Deep Rest

Non-sleep deep rest (also known as NSDR) is a resting mind state that can significantly increase your neuroplasticity and enhance your brain's ability to create new, positive neural connections. A good way to enter this mind state is by using mind-body practices that cultivate it, including any form of yoga nidra (otherwise known as "sleeping yoga") or any type of body scan. Both are resting practices in which you start by lying on your back and allow yourself to be guided, as you dreamily follow along. The important thing is that the practice you choose is narrated by someone, whether you're in a class, on Zoom, or listening to a recording. This relieves your mind from the effort of trying to focus your attention (as one does in meditation, by returning to a primary focal point, such as the breath, a mantra, or simply the present moment itself). Most practices last for twenty to thirty minutes.

In yoga nidra, you first set an intention (or *sankalpa*) to guide your practice. Then you follow a teacher's guided visualization, allowing your mind to quiet its thinking and planning and to become conscious of the sensations of aliveness that emanate from your body—including parts of the body you might not often think about, like the inside of your cheek, the back of your tongue, the tip of your tongue, the tip of your nose, your jaw. From here, you move on to focus on larger body areas of which these small areas are a part, such as your head. Eventually, your focus encompasses your whole body. The goal in yoga nidra is to engage not just your mind but your whole being on a more intangible level.

Happily, there are many free and excellent yoga nidra teachings online. Ally Boothroyd, Lizzy Hill, and Kamini Desai offer highly regarded practices, which they've made available online. Boothroyd, whose online practices vary in length from twenty minutes to an hour, likens yoga nidra to "a full-body massage for your brain and entire peripheral nervous system" to help you "drop into the deepest states of rest and relaxation." For a *sankalpa*, she suggests setting the intention of "I rest deeply to honor and restore each layer of myself," which you mentally whisper to yourself three times. Or you might use an affirmation as your *sankalpa*—"I am loved," "I am healing," "I am at peace"—whatever affirmation or intention resonates with you or delivers the message you most need to hear.

When I practice yoga nidra, shifting my focus to the incoming stream of sensations from my body, often for the first time that day, I feel that I'm in direct contact with my body's aliveness in a very intimate and receptive way. And that brings me back into, well, my life force. My thought stream slows until my thoughts have dissipated into nothingness. My whole being quiets, and I melt into something larger, something safe, something primordial. And when I emerge, I carry that sense of expansiveness with me. Small irritations and difficult people who might normally get my goat don't. I'm more awake to the beauty of everything.

Practicing a body scan is another way to enter a non-sleep deep rest state. Here, too, you focus on different parts of the body, but the goal is a little different: to notice sensations of physical tightness or pent-up tension and release that tension. A favorite of mine, which I have over the years memorized and use almost every night before I fall asleep (and reemploy when I wake up in the middle of the night and worries swoop in, as worries will), is Jon Kabat-Zinn's classic Mindfulness-Based Stress Reduction Body Scan, of which you can find various iterations wherever you download your music or on YouTube. One aside here: If you, too, find your ruminations swoop in on you when you wake up at 3:00 A.M., you're not alone—research shows that three-quarters of individuals say they are most likely to ruminate at night. (As one of the characters in Sigrid Nunez's novel *The Vulnerables* says, "Insomnia is the inability to forget.") NSDR is a great antidote to nighttime mind drama, too.

Research confirms that when we can achieve this interior sensation of aliveness within stillness, it's extremely good for us. When you practice NSDR, for example, your thought stream does slow down dramatically; you go from having thirty-five thoughts per minute to one to three thoughts per minute. Meanwhile, your blood pressure goes down and your body slows its production of inflammatory stress hormones. Feel-good, healthy hormones that make us happy to be here, happy to get to live this life, like dopamine and oxytocin, increase. And if you get this kind of deep rest right after working at learning something new, like a new language or a piece of music, or memorizing the lines of a presentation, your rate of retention significantly increases.

Floating

Here's another approach to true rest—though it includes getting wet. Researchers at the Laureate Institute for Brain Research have found that spending time in a sensory deprivation, or floating, tank—without external stimuli or stimulation—

can "reset the nervous system, signaling the default mode network to reboot and relax." For those of us who have trouble resting on our own, it can help to have this time imposed upon us. (In an era in which our nervous systems are constantly being bombarded by sensory chaos and overload, this includes all of us.) Floating in a sensory deprivation tank—in salt water, in the dark—is a balm to the nervous system, allowing your brain and body to fully, truly relax.

But if that feels like too much, and you are a competent swimmer, try this hack: Float on your back in a nearby pool, or better yet, the salty sea, or a lake (if weather allows). Floating on your back, staring up at the sky, while your body is buoyant, frees the mind to let go while opening up your senses. As someone who grew up on the Chesapeake Bay, I know this to be true: Floating and ruminating simply cannot happen at the same time.

Mindfulness—Of Course!

We can't talk about rest and quiet without also talking about mindfulness and meditation. As a regular meditator, I profoundly believe in and have reaped its many benefits. I can't start my day without it. (I'm so wedded to it as a life skill, I once wrote a book largely about the science of meditation.) I credit my daily twenty minutes of morning meditation for making me kinder and more patient with my friends, my family, and myself (at least after twenty years, I certainly hope it has). My mindfulness training has no doubt helped me find layers of relief from overidentifying with my emotions, memories, or thoughts during some of the most difficult moments of my life. In this way, it is an excellent prophylactic for rumination.

The goal of any mindfulness practice is to use your volition to shift your attention from aimless mental chatter to present-moment attention, often by using a focal point (such as your breath, or the sensation of your belly filling with air, or the sounds around you), to help ground you while allowing yourself to accept whatever arises within you. Even if your mind wanders away over and over again, that's okay; it's refocusing your attention that matters. The payoff can be profound. In one study of twenty-three male combat veterans, those who underwent mindfulness-based interventions showed healthy changes in neural connectivity in the default mode network, compared to a control group. This, in turn, helped veterans to increase their ability to move out of the unwanted thoughts that threatened to pull them back into painful, traumatic memories and rumination. So, even as I think it should go without saying, I'll say it here anyway: The more meditation—of any type—the better.

You can take meditation classes, of course, or download a meditation app. There are many to choose from. Because I love to meditate, I have four apps on my phone: Calm, Headspace, Waking Up, and Dharma Seed (the latter is free and full of thousands of excellent meditations by leading teachers, including two of my favorites, Tara Brach and Sylvia Boorstein).

One powerful meditation I often return to is called the Wheel of Awareness, which was created by Dan Siegel, MD. The Wheel of Awareness is an excellent tool to help you practice mindful awareness and is unusual in that it includes three powerful types of mindfulness: focused attention, open awareness, and kind intention, which, Siegel has shown, can lead to greater calm, insight, and emotional regulation, and enhance neural connections. (You can find many versions of Siegel's Wheel of Awareness online.)

One caveat here: In perusing the research on rumination, I've learned that meditation in and of itself may not be enough to train our brains out of our rumination habits. Moreover, for some people, according to Ruth Lanius, "it worsens their thought loops, taking them further into rumination, rather than helping them escape it." It's a crucial tool in the healing toolbox, without question. But since "no one approach works for everyone," Lanius advises, "it makes good sense to add in other modalities and practical strategies to help you move out of rumination." But if it feels right for you and doesn't worsen your thought loops, I highly recommend you make meditation one of your chosen strategies.

However we come to it, pure rest can be one of our antiruminative modalities. When Sam talks about needing more stillness, more rest, more alone time, he's voicing his longing for something that is deeply restorative, allowing his default mode network to lower its burden and bring him back into a sense of connection with his core self. For so many of us, rumination is what is keeping us from self-realization. And self-realization is, ultimately, what we are all going for, isn't it? If we can achieve that renewed sense of self from actions that don't require much effort but the very opposite—deep rest—all the better.

TWELVE

When You Need More Help

I WOULD LIKE to tell you that everything I've learned about ruminating, and about how to move beyond it, has made me rumination-proof. I am not and perhaps never will be. For that to be true, I would have to have had a less arduous coming-of-age experience and fewer serious health problems. Nonetheless, over the past year, I have seen measurable progress—as the evidence later in this chapter will show. We will never stop having challenges, and if we do the work, we will never stop growing in response to them, which is part of what gives such grandeur to the life journey that each of us must take.

The struggle is, in its own way, a gift (not that it seems that way at the time, of course—far from it). In all my years of interviewing individuals from every kind of background, and leading thinkers in so many different fields, I've seen over and over again that the more pain someone has known, the more curious, creative, and self-realized that person often becomes over time. When we have known suffering, we are, I think, offered a choice to embark on something of a hero's journey—a truth that stands at the heart of every bildungsroman and young adult novel, from *The Lord of the Rings* to *A Tree Grows in Brooklyn.* And on that hero's journey, the only viable option, if we hope to inhabit a realized life, is to forge new paths that call to us.

If you were never shown the blueprint for how to live an unbroken, emotionally connected, and meaningful life, you must design that for yourself. If you accept this challenge, you will, by the very nature of the process, undergo a dramatic change within yourself and in how you meet the world. But as you undertake your journey, you must be willing to revisit your whole story and greet and love all the aspects of yourself you meet along the way.

This is the work we have been doing here, together. And it's the work that I must continue to do, because I see now that there are aspects of my story that still warrant attention. You, too, may be feeling both the gladness of transmuting your ruminations into something insightful and hopeful, and the realization that there are still emotional triggers—activating events—that destabilize you.

I've worked through many of the activating conditions that have given rise to my stickiest ruminations. And I see—ever-more clearly—why the incident with the British researcher was so upsetting for me. It was an echo, even if a very faint one, of so many situations, from childhood on, when people in authority—men in power, and at times, even my mother, lost in her own grief and pain—dismissed me and my feelings. But what the work I've done has also enabled me to see is the link between my mother's experience and my own. My mother's world, in a single year of her life, changed unalterably with the death of my father, which was arguably the direct result of a medical error. He'd gone in for minor GI surgery, but when he complained to my mother of severe pain after the operation and asked her to get the surgeon to come, the surgeon refused. When he was paged, he was playing golf and told the nurse to tell my mother, "Pain after surgery is normal." But this was not normal pain; it was terrible pain from internal bleeding, and it went unrecognized. So my father developed peritonitis, went into septic shock, and died.

No one had believed my mother, the worried young wife—the hysteric—that something was not right.

Years later, I had a similar experience with my son, who was born with a rare disorder that, if not caught, most babies die from within the first few weeks of life. He was projectile vomiting every day, so every day, I went to the office of our pediatrician to find out what was wrong. Each time, he patted me on the back and handed me another pamphlet: one on maternal anxiety; another on postpartum depression; another on colic. Finally, the female pediatrician who owned the practice saw me in the waiting room for the third day in a row. She asked me what was wrong, why I kept coming back, and something spilled out of my mouth like, "My baby can't nurse and when he does he vomits it all up and he's in pain and something's not right. . . . I feel it in my bones . . . something's not right with my baby." And I burst into tears; of course I did. She took us into an exam room, closed the door, gently palpated my son's belly, and within ten minutes had called a surgeon at Hopkins with whom she'd gone to medical school. That surgeon (who, like my neurologist, and hematologist, and cardiologist, is a lovely, lovely man, so I am not trying to portray all male doctors as misogynists) saved my son's life. But had I believed what I was being told—that I was the problem, just another woman with postpartum anxiety or depression—for even another forty-eight hours, my son would probably have died as so many babies with his condition do.

It took me a long time to understand how experiences like the ones my mother and I both went through, at the hands of men who refused to listen to us because they saw us as hysterical, shaped the way we moved through the world. My mother and I have both known what it is to be unheard—to speak and find our words dismissed, as if seeing a coming danger and naming it with emotion, were itself a flaw. In a culture that so often sees women's voices as not worth listening to, it's easy to internalize the message that what we say will never matter. The result is a kind of silence that seeps in slowly and persistently. Reclaiming my voice is even now a work in progress. There is clearly a layer of wounding that I have not yet attended to. If I am to reclaim my voice, I'm going to have to sit with old wounds, notice where that fear still lingers in my body, and honor the parts of myself that have yet to be fully heard and seen—by me.

You might not have a story of adversity like mine (and I hope you don't), but whether your experiences are more severe or less, you almost certainly have some history that has called you to be here. Perhaps, as I do, you recognize that even with your newly honed practices, when circumstances and triggers collide in a particularly toxic alchemy, the tools you've developed to quell your mind drama are still insufficient to do the job.

The skills we have practiced together here have transformed my life, and I hope they have transformed yours. But for those moments when I still find myself spinning out of control, I'm like an ice skater with the twisties, gyrating in space, unable to orient my mind and body so that I can stick my landing. Yes, I need more help.

Some of Us Have Met with More Suffering Than Others

For each of us, what tips us over into the kind of rumination that has the potential to immobilize us is different. This includes many factors in addition to growing up with early adversity. Below is by no means a comprehensive list of those factors, some of which may resonate with experiences of your own.

Grown-Up Trauma. What triggers you into rumination you seem unable to escape might not have happened when you were young but during the years of accumulated losses after childhood. The bad things that shouldn't have happened to you but did. The spouse who cheated on you. The right life partner you haven't yet found. The recognition you were due, but didn't receive, while others did. A sexual assault. Sometimes the worst things that happen to us come later in life—the devastating divorce, the medical diagnosis, the near loss or loss of a child, the car accident, the fire that swept away much of what we hold dear. Any or all of these things may tip us into that ruminative state that is so all-consuming. Multiple studies show that the degree to which we ruminate after traumatic life events predicts whether we will develop a more intractable form of rumination: PTSD.

Growing Up Female. Susan Nolen-Hoeksema at Yale was the first researcher to find that women tend to ruminate more than men; 57 percent of women are, she wrote, "immobilized by overthinking," compared to 43 percent of men. This gender difference emerges in early adolescence and persists into adulthood, with girls and women reporting higher levels of rumination than boys and men. This is part of the reason why, Nolen-Hoeksema argued, women suffer from depression at twice the rate of men. More recent research in neuroscience has shown that she was right. Due to differences in how the female brain processes stress, compared to the male brain, women are more likely to "act in" on ourselves, turning on ourselves in self-judgment—which is, as we've learned, linked to a greater likelihood of depression. Men, on the other hand, are more likely to "act out" in behavior.

But it's impossible to separate biology from biography. Women grow up internalizing the misogynistic voices directed against us; fuel for self-derogatory rumination. (Perhaps this is why many women I interviewed often found themselves ruminating about the things men said or did that diminished them, and their difficulty in voicing themselves in response.) Women also have to move through the world differently due to the threat of violence; females are statistically more likely to suffer the traumas of sexual, verbal, and emotional abuse, which helps explain why so many women develop depression, anxiety disorders, and PTSD. "I lost all sense of myself" is a feeling women report again and again in response to these experiences.

Structural Racism and Marginalization. Structural racism, poverty, and discrimination are all experiences encoded with false messages of non-belonging. For BIPOC Americans, growing up with the threat of racism; facing discrimination, poverty, or community violence; living in a food-insecure household; going to substandard schools; lacking adequate housing; and often being given substandard medical care (if any)—all these experiences reinforce the messaging of otherness and non-belonging. The same is true for the marginalization and sometimes downright vilification of those who identify as LGBTQ. The more you are targeted, demeaned, or deprived of respect and equality, the harder it is to know you belong. The harder it is to know you matter.

Chronic Illness. To some degree, we all fall into moments of existential fear and rumination about the inevitability of our death. That said, when there has been a history of family medical crises or we have struggled from long-standing health concerns, we will inevitably ruminate more about our health. (I certainly fall into this category.) Brain scans show that in individuals with chronic conditions, the area of the default mode network that should help us with healthy interoception—the area that gives us valuable information about how our bodies are feeling—can become hypervigilant, mistaking harmless sensations for indications that something serious is wrong.

Researchers who examine the relationship between rumination and illness have reiterated this; in one study, rumination led to not only the intensification of physical symptoms but poorer clinical health outcomes. Happily, study after study also shows that targeting rumination, and emotional pain, in order to treat chronic pain, yields a powerful and beneficial effect.

Post-Traumatic Stress Disorder. When there has been a history of very severe abuse or trauma, as in PTSD, the default mode network can (as I alluded to in the footnote in chapter 5) behave differently. Instead of becoming hyperactive and firing on all cylinders on a closed loop, unable to sync up to the rest of the brain, activity in the default mode network drops off to the point that it kind of loses power, like an engine without enough gas. Individuals may feel numb, checked out, and not really alive. Lanius explains, "Individuals with severe trauma may feel dissociated from what's going on around them. Often, they can't access their sense of self at all." And when this is the case, it's crucial to work directly with a trauma-informed practitioner to get the help and relief you so deeply deserve.

I share the above with you not to generalize or categorize your experience and truth. I simply want to offer you the validation that your story of loss, or injustice, or suffering is legitimate. It matters, as do you.

Healing from Trauma

This is not a book about PTSD or early life trauma. Still, as someone who feels I am only now dealing with what I was never before willing to label as trauma—nobody beat me when I was a child, sexually abused me, locked me in a closet, bombed my family's home and left us homeless—I now understand that at least some forms of trauma don't look dramatic from the outside. Those forms of trauma are more about what a practitioner I worked with (whom you'll soon meet) described as "an absence of presence." This feels like a good moniker for what I have been feeling over the past year while investigating my own sources of rumination and the best means of healing from them.

Perhaps no one knows more about how to solidify the gains we've made in tending to our oldest wounds than Ruth Lanius. As head of a major research center, she is intimately aware of the array of modalities just emerging from the field of neuroscience to address the grip trauma can have on our mental acts.

"What modalities do you find most exciting right now—what holds the most promise in your survey of the research?" I ask during one of our monthly Zoom calls.

Lanius tells me about a recent study she did with colleagues to assess the efficacy of a mind-body therapy called *Deep Brain Reorienting*, or DBR, which targets the brain stem. "The results are some of the most exciting I've seen in the body of research I've done in my career."

The words *most exciting* certainly grab my attention. So do the words *mind* and *body*, which suggest that this modality addresses not just the mind but somatic sensations in the body. It was only a few months earlier that Mark Trullinger had shown me on a brain scan the extreme reaction I had to the word *somatic* and suggested that working with sensations in my body would be crucial to resolving my stickiest wounds and the ruminations they fuel.

When the pain of trauma is felt, Lanius explains, "it is first experienced in your brain stem, at the base of your brain." You might think of your brain stem as your brain's foundation—like the foundation of your house or apartment building. It is here, in the brain stem, that "you first experience the shock of trauma as it is happening to you. And that shock response is felt in your body even before emotional processing occurs." This is true whether something traumatic occurs when you are in the womb or at age ninety-two.

This is the first therapy I have ever heard of, I tell Lanius, that focuses on the role of the brain stem in healing. Until very recently, the brain stem has been viewed as a primitive brain hub of little therapeutic consequence and thus largely ignored when it comes to emotional health. Interest in the brain stem first arose when psychiatrist Frank Corrigan, MD, who specializes in the neurobiology of trauma, and practices and trains other psychologists in the United Kingdom, developed a protocol that goes directly to the brain stem to address the shock of trauma where, he contends, it is first experienced.

"What does the brain look like when the brain stem has been impacted by trauma?" I ask Lanius.

"There is a lack of healthy integration." Over Zoom, Lanius shows me what this looks like on brain scans. One can see numerous areas in which it looks like someone has sketched very faint, barely visible blue lines rising from the base of the brain. These lines, she explains, demonstrate "a lack of healthy brain connectivity between the brain stem and the rest of the brain." Higher up in these same brain scans, Lanius shows me what look like bright red clusters of dots—blobs, really. These red areas indicate unhealthy overactivity higher up in the brain. Taken together, these scans, Lanius tells me, show "a lack of vertical integration in the brain; the brain is not connecting up from the brain stem into the thinking brain in the way we want it to."

In a separate 2023 randomized controlled trial, Lanius and Corrigan demonstrated that patients who underwent just eight sessions of DBR showed significant reductions in symptoms of PTSD. Lanius believes patients experience such profound improvements with DBR because it helps to repair neural connections and create healthier neural integration between the brain stem and the rest of the brain. She is setting out to investigate this question now.

"How does all this relate to our default mode network and our ruminations?" I ask Lanius.

"Unless we deal with and clear that initial shock lodged in the brain stem, we can't resolve the unprocessed traumatic experiences and emotions that play a role in triggering rumination," she underscores. For the nerds among us, what might this look like on a neuroanatomical level? The brain stem is a stalklike structure at the base of your brain—part of what Lanius calls your *survival brain.* Your survival brain also includes structures known as the *periaqueductal gray,* or PAG, and the *locus coeruleus,* or LC. When you are, for lack of a better word, triggered, your brain stem, PAG, and LC generate and send raw, unprocessed vibrations of shock and emotion up from the base of your skull. This shock reverberates throughout your brain. Unless you are trained to register it, this vibrational tone remains far below your conscious awareness. But your nervous system does register it, as your brain stem sends these shock reverberations up into higher levels of your brain—what Lanius terms your *emotional learning brain*—which includes your hippocampus and amygdala. And these areas, in turn, send that potent vibrational shock energy upstream into your *reflective brain*—yup, right into your default mode network. The result is those feelings of fear and dismay that suddenly flood you.

As Lanius explains to me, this is why, once the shock stored in the brain stem is addressed, "patients say they feel safer. . . . It's because we've changed those intense visceral feelings. And this allows them to reevaluate who they are and how they interact with the world."

By addressing the brain stem, it becomes possible for the rest of your brain, including your default mode network, to experience less fear, less rumination, in the face of the kinds of stressors that are most likely to trigger you. Even when you experience situations that closely echo the old hurt—so close you almost flinch—you notice you can stand back a little now. You find, to your own surprise, a small circle of safety and well-being inside yourself, and it holds.

Am I game to give this a try? Of course I am. And so I commit to eight sessions with psychologist Jessica Christie-Sands, PhD, who coauthored Frank Corrigan's first research paper on

DBR and trains others in DBR. Before we begin, she explains a bit about the kind of early life trauma that DBR helps to process. As children, we are primed to orient ourselves toward connection. It is our lifeline. "But when we turn toward our parent and that parent is present, but absent, we are met with the painful presence of absence." And "when you don't have connection, it's really hard to form healthy attachment. This might mean you didn't get to experience an early sense of safety." As a child, this lack of connection and the safety that comes with connection is registered as a shock in the brain stem. It is shocking as an infant or child to find you have no one to turn to. That shock "interferes with our sense of belonging." Without that sense of belonging, we don't know how to hold on to our own sense of our presence, of who we are; we experience a disruption in self-location, in self-orienting. And as a result, we have trouble orienting ourselves in our surroundings—in literal time and space.

This resonates with me. As a preteen and teenager, I had very little sense of where I was in space and time. (Perhaps this is why everyone called me a space cadet?) I was the klutz, ever the laughingstock, the one with two left feet. I sometimes struggled, embarrassingly, even to remember which side was left and which was right. When I tried aerobics when I first landed in New York in the 1980s, I was hopeless. All the other students would zag left and I would zag right. Even today, in physical therapy, my therapist will say, "Lift your left arm." I'll lift my right, and she'll say, "Lift your *other* left," and we will laugh. I just thought that was me, my clumsy inadequacy. It certainly never occurred to me that it might be related to the early shock of trauma, lodged deep in the recesses of my brain stem.

Finally, Christie-Sands tells me, when you find there is no one to turn to as a child, you may learn to "become compliant before you try to attach. Your system might also learn to reduce your visibility. If, as you turn toward another person, you can't safely orient toward them, or if, as you try to connect, there is a punishing component to your interactions, or you are taught to flinch with self-blame, then you learn to become invisible to mitigate the threat and feel safe."

DBR: Whispering to the Deepest Part of the Brain

How does DBR address the early shock still lingering in our brains? Christie-Sands begins each session by asking me to recall a moment from something that's "upper level" in my mind, an event fresh from the pages of my recent life—as recent as a few hours ago—that really activated me. Usually, she explains, it is recent moments in which we felt triggered that allow us to access the shock mapped into our brain stems from earlier in our lives. "We do this by turning toward the moment—the feelings, the words—of that shock state and slowly learning how to safely reorient ourselves as we experience the sensations of stored shock and allow them to dissipate."

Because this is a whole-body experience, I didn't take notes during our sessions—that would have interfered with the emotional and somatic processing—so what follows are mere glimpses of what I remember experiencing. Here's how our sessions were structured: For the first twenty-five minutes, we talked until we homed in on a recent activating event—something I'd found myself struggling to let go of.

After we identified that, Christie-Sands helped me to orient myself in the room by closing my eyes and making a mental map of the walls, the space, the sounds, the light around me.

Once I was oriented in time and space, she helped me to go into my body and experience the feelings that arose from my activating event, focusing on the sensations that were coming from my brain stem—pain and tension at the back of my head, in my neck, across my forehead, behind my eyes, along my shoulders. The sensations I experienced at the beginning of my first session were very intense, but with each session that followed, I could feel more and more as if something were loosening and dissipating—another layer of shock energy. What follows are descriptions of the sensations, and the unexpected emotional states they give rise to, at their most intense.

ONE

Chills up my spine. Words flit through my mind, that old, cold feeling: *No one is there.* My body starts to shake uncontrollably—the shakes one has after childbirth, or a surgery in the hospital, or a car accident. The freezing cold in my spine rises into my head, my body shaking, shuddering with the chill. Body rocking involuntarily. Pain rising in my throat, so painful, as if my voice is being choked off. I hear myself repeating, "No one is there." I feel the emptiness all around me. I am sobbing. And yet in this moment, as I listen to Christie-Sands's voice gently coaching me, I turn toward that pain, I hold the pain. I am surrounded by it and yet safely holding that pain within myself. I am able to be with, be witness to, this shock energy, these waves of reverberating pain. Slowly, it subsides. I hold it. I turn toward it. My body stills. I breathe deeply. Something feels changed.

TWO

Quivering breath. Ears ringing. Pain behind eyes. A hollowing below my ribs. The dread that fills that hollow, drumming cavity I feel myself to be. Head pounding. *No one is coming,* I hear in my head. Pain pounding at the base of my skull, moving up through my neck and jaw, tightening around my forehead in the old vise I know so well. *No one wants to hear what you have to say!* The shame I feel. The old humiliation. Hunching down as if protecting my shoulders from blows. The shock of not being met with care or comfort in my most vulnerable moments. Of being made fun of. The tightness around my throat. Too painful to swallow. Too painful to talk. Waves of shuddering. They come again. And again. And again. Sobbing. Such sobbing. Sobbing that feels endless. Then, sitting with the shuddering. Welcoming myself to myself, whatever comes. Holding on to my sense of belonging after the shuddering. The part of me that knows I do belong.

THREE

Huge waves of pain at the back of my skull. Fire-hot poker behind my eyes. Words swim through my mind: *Leave me alone! What did I ever do? Stop! Stop!* My body is goosenecking, folding into itself, ducking. Squeezing my eyes shut. Bracing myself. More waves of pain. Tears. Waves. Shock waves. More tension, rising from deep in my skull, my spine. Such sadness. So much sadness. Sadness everywhere. Sobs. Sitting with this. Holding myself in this. Then: "I see you. I've got you." Who is speaking? Me. I am talking to me. I am soothing myself. The tenderness starts flooding in, intermingling with the sadness. I put my hands instinctively over my heart. I feel more like . . . I am me. More of a sense of me-ness. I feel present—with myself.

FOUR

The old tension in my forehead, spine, at the back of my head. Small pockets of cold rising in my spine, up from my bones, from my very cells. Silent shudders. Then not so silent. Quaking. Shuddering. Pulsing. Vibrating into tears. I hear the words "I have to pull myself back from death, alone." So many times. Scenes of being in the hospital at five, fourteen, twenty-nine. Blood transfusions. Heart procedures. The hospital at thirty-six, forty-two, forty-four. Again, at forty-seven, forty-nine. The ambulance rides. The long, long hospital stays. The time I coded. The terror of every minute of it. The freezing chill of every hospital room. The waves of pain. Shaking. Quaking. *You have to pull yourself from death, alone* keeps repeating in my head. Sitting with the fear. Holding my pain. Holding me. Holding this body. The words shortening until I hear: *Death, alone.* I sit with each pocket of cold as it rises, allowing it to come up and through me. More waves—tears, shaking? They are indistinguishable. Then, slowly, small waves of heat. At last, a warmth spreading up my spine. My body expanding. Breath widening. A centeredness. New, unexpected words arise: *How extraordinary that you, alone, pulled yourself from death.* Shame at being in the wrong body, the sick body, becomes . . . grace. Yes, grace. Pain's antithesis. Spine tingling with warmth, I feel myself, my groundedness. I feel myself grow bigger, enlarging to fill the space around me. *I am here. I am here.*

These sessions brought about potent changes for me. I am, I think, uncovering a layer of my story that lies beyond my conscious awareness—one that is visceral, somatic, and true. After our first eight sessions, the effects were so powerful that I decided to do four more. As I tell Christie-Sands, "I feel like I've been looking for this all my life, to feel this grounded, alive, rooted, my feet planted under me. And I've been wondering what's wrong with me that, despite all the work I've done, I couldn't find it."

On a practical level, I am more aware of my agitation when it arises, and as a result, I get less juiced up. My capacity to handle difficult moments or interactions that touch into very old wounds is indeed greater, and the threshold for what triggers my rumination is much higher. Perhaps this is because when circumstances or people prove difficult, I am better able to orient myself into right here, where life is happening, without having to turn away, subjugate my needs, or camouflage myself. Things feel clearer, more manageable. I'm quicker to speak up, too, because I'm able to tap into my voice and wisdom faster, with more clarity, than before. The biggest gain is this: I feel less afraid. So I ruminate less. It feels good.

I touch base with Ruth Lanius about my progress with DBR. My gains "make sense," she says. "Your brain stem is no longer hijacking your brain. You're addressing those lower survival levels that still affect raw arousal, and as a result, your default mode network is no longer driven by threat. By repairing the foundation, you are repairing the first floor and the second floor. You can finally heal."

Home-Use Gadgets to Stop Rumination

We are entering a neurotechnology renaissance in healthcare, so I would be remiss if I didn't touch briefly on home-use gadgets now available on the marketplace. In the past several years, the field of neurotechnology has exploded with FDA-approved home devices and nifty new gadgets, some of which have been shown to help rewire the default mode network in healthy and constructive ways. A recent survey in the journal *Brain Stimulation* found over a thousand clinical trials using a neuromodulation treatment for home use, to treat overall well-being, as well as depression and memory loss.

These home devices aren't for everyone, but if you love a good tech hack, they might appeal to you. I began trialing them about two-thirds of the way into my journey to transform my rumination into something more purposeful. Used together with the many approaches we've learned, they have the potential to help solidify your gains. That said, before using any devices, please check with your doctor. Some may require a prescription—or at the very least, a thumbs-up from a healthcare professional who knows your history and your needs.

After surveying several leading neuroscientists and psychiatrists, I landed on two devices for me.

The DAVID Delight Pro by Mind Alive is a portable, relatively affordable FDA-cleared device that comes with goggles, earphones, and ear-stimulation clips, and allows you to safely do home sessions of neurostimulation, which can help improve attention, mood, and memory. It has a setting for cranial electrical stimulation (CES), which is exactly that: electrical stimulation to your cranium. I used the DAVID Delight Pro for three months. I found it easy to use, and though it was hard to put my finger on any single change, it left me feeling calmer and more centered. I liked it so much for its calming effects that I gave it to one of my children.

There are many other FDA-cleared devices like the DAVID Delight Pro that help address a variety of symptoms, including anxiety, and that also offer cranial electrical stimulation.

Some of the most commonly used devices include the Alpha-Stim (which uses ear clips for electrode placement); the Fisher Wallace Stimulator (which uses sponge electrodes placed on the temples); the Cervella Cranial Electrotherapy Stimulator, specifically for anxiety and insomnia (which delivers micro pulses of electric current via electrodes in the ear cushions of the headset); the CES Ultra (which uses electrodes on the temples); and the MINDGear CES (which allows you to choose between using ear clips or self-adhesive electrodes for the temples).

Instead of getting a new electrical stimulation device for myself (much as I liked the DAVID Delight Pro), I decided to upgrade to a much more expensive device that many of my friends who are neuroscientists use, the Vielight Neuro Gamma. In my 2020 book, *The Angel and the Assassin,* I reported on research at MIT showing that pulsing LED lights directly into the default mode network at a frequency of 40 hertz—safely and from outside the head—helped significantly with mental clarity, memory, and attention. At the time, I'd been fascinated by this promising marriage between neuroscience and technology. Five years later, a similar 40 hertz gamma light-delivery technology is now available to all through a company called Vielight. After trying the Vielight gamma device for three months, I felt I was better able to find that word right on the tip of my tongue and to remember that I'd let the dog out and where I'd put my keys. Suddenly, I was reminded of how my brain worked when I was much younger. Of course, what I was experiencing may also be part of the consolidation of gains from my yearslong journey to quell my ruminations and turn them into something purposeful and empowering. Hard to say. But it was significant enough that I felt more confident. That said, we do know that neural healing is always multifactorial. The more we do to assist the brain toward neural integration, the more it does for us in return.

My experience aligned with the research. In a 2024 study, researchers showed that when the Vielight's LED lights were positioned on the default mode network, the 40 hertz gamma frequency helped to enhance cognitive functioning; creative, divergent thinking; and idea generation. I asked Lew Lim, PhD, Vielight's founder, and the inventor of the devices the company sells, how the gamma light fuels better memory and more fluid creative thought. He explained to me, "If you inhibit the default mode network and move on to other networks, you release the brain to perform better and get enhanced creativity." In layperson terms, when we prevent the default mode network from becoming overactive and coax it to connect to the whole brain, we reap significant benefits in how we think and feel.

(The Vielight devices are not inexpensive. In full disclosure, I was gifted one for trial use by the company. But my experience was notable enough that when a friend decided she needed one, too, I bought one for myself and gave mine to her.)

Not a Device but a Drug

There is one other approach I wanted to try—but didn't. I'm still waiting for FDA approval to work up my nerve. But you might—as long as, again, you check first with a healthcare professional to see if it's the right choice for you. Psilocybin has been shown to decrease rumination while simultaneously increasing creative flow in a way traditional treatments do not. A 2022 study by researchers at the University of California San Francisco looked at whether psilocybin could be as powerful as the SSRI Lexapro (escitalopram) in treating unhealthy rumination over a six-week period. Participants using low-dose psilocybin showed significantly less rumination—but psilocybin came with an added benefit: It did not suppress study participants' creative thoughts the way the SSRI did. Those on Lexapro showed a decrease in rumination but also reported "thought suppression" and a loss of "psychological insight." Psilocybin, on the other hand, decreased unhealthy rumination while also opening the brain for creative thought and deeper layers of self-awareness. A 2023 study showed that using psychedelics altered connectivity in the default mode network, increasing "functional connectivity" between the default mode and the rest of the brain.

MDMA (commonly known as Ecstasy) has similarly been shown, when administered under proper supervision, to be a powerful psychotherapeutic intervention. It creates changes in the default mode network, helping to bring forth positive memories, while rendering negative memories as less negative. Ketamine has also been shown to create changes in the default mode network in ways that help to lessen individuals' hypervigilance.

There are, of course, other science-based ways to help individuals heal from PTSD and developmental trauma. According to Lanius, these include neurofeedback (the promising effects of which I have experienced myself; over the past decade, I've undergone two courses of neurofeedback, and each time, it's been like getting a tune-up for my brain); prolonged exposure therapy; somatic experiencing; Eye Movement Desensitization and Reprocessing (EMDR); and trauma-based cognitive behavioral therapy. All of these, she tells me, have shown promise in "helping individuals to overcome the timeless nature of traumatic memories, increase emotional awareness, and reclaim bodily awareness by improving the function of the default mode network."

Wherever you find yourself on your journey, if your past carries the weight of trauma and your heart calls for more support, honor that quiet voice. You are, and always have been, worthy of care. When you step toward the healing you deserve, you may even discover a deeper love for your own story and a wellspring of compassion for yourself—proof that even our deepest and most enduring struggles can, over time, lead us somewhere luminous.

IV

Spiral Up!

THIRTEEN

The Upside of Rumination

"YOU ONLY HAVE one mind and you'll live in it the rest of your life, so make sure it's a nice place to live." I heard one of my favorite writers, Pulitzer Prize–winning author Marilynne Robinson, say this recently in an interview with *The New York Times*'s Ezra Klein. Robinson tells the story of how, when she was in high school, a teacher told her this, and that single statement "had a bigger effect on me than anything else anyone ever said to me."

We are all looking for ways to make our minds that nicer place to inhabit, and Robinson has certainly found her path there by writing extraordinary fiction. We might not have her gifts, but I believe we all can, each in our own way, find the upside of rumination and navigate to a more creative and fulfilling life—"a nice place to live." In some ways, this is what we've been preparing for throughout this journey: to arrive at the doorway of a more expansive kind of mind-wandering that enriches rather than contains and stifles us, where the same expenditure of mental energy that fuels our negative ruminations can, instead, power a transformation that enhances our lives.

Earlier, I quoted *Merriam-Webster*'s definition of *ruminate*, which focused on the negative aspect we've been discussing until now, the going over the same matter in one's mind "repeatedly" with little "purposive thinking." But to quote more of *Merriam-Webster*'s definition, there is an upside: to "engage in contemplation," and to "reflect." Synonyms for *ruminate* include to "ponder" and to "muse." *Ruminate* is a word—and an act—that contains within itself a duality. It can encompass both the light and the dark sides of a "seriously" thinking mind: brooding versus self-reflection; replaying past wounds, mistakes, regrets, and old conflicts versus introspection that leads to ahas, insights, and new choices; obsessing over feelings of failure versus using those past experiences to pivot to new ideas; self-flagellation versus making meaning out of what happened to you in ways that will shape a very different, and more joyful, future.

One of the best case studies I know of to illustrate this upside concerns a man I will call Armand. Born in New York of an American mother and a French father, Armand grew up as an expat in Lyon; his father was a physics professor at a French university. Armand followed in his father's footsteps, though in a different field of study and in his home country; he now teaches European history at a small liberal arts college in the Midwest. Armand is thirty-five years old. His hair is a study in chaos—dark, curly, and untamed—setting off the clarity of his light, wide-set eyes. There is a premature gravity to him, as if an unnameable weight has settled on his tall frame. Not in the way of the perpetually anxious but in the way of someone who carries something unspoken on his mind. It's because of that, perhaps, that Armand has been curious about the work I'm doing around rumination and how it clouds our more creative, clear-minded selves.

Recently, Armand came up for tenure. He was, he tells me, "caught in that vise of rumination, and its screws kept turning tighter." He'd always thought that if he finally achieved academia's holy grail, he'd know relief and maybe even earn his father's respect at last. But when he was finally given the good news, the "reprieve from trepidation, from waiting and worrying, was so momentary, I realized I was never going to escape my self-loathing, not really. Not unless I did something proactive."

"Can you take me inside your head, that mental vise you spoke of, before and after you got tenure?" I ask. "What does that rumination sound and feel like?"

Armand deliberates for a moment. Sadness flicks its fin in his gray eyes before he voices his darker thoughts. *What makes you think* you're *worthy of tenure? You're only thirty-five; you have friends who are a lot more talented than you are and they still don't have tenure. Your work is no better than theirs. And what if your department knew how often you procrastinate? What if they knew how often you worry you have nothing new to say? Sure, you've published a bit, but you and I both know you have nothing truly important to contribute in your supposed area of 'expertise.' Not really. Yeah, you're pretty much full of it. And what happens when you have to take on a leadership role in your department? Plan conferences? Be department chair? Do you* really *think you have that kind of good judgment? What happens when you screw it all up, as you probably will? You'll be a drag on the department. They'll figure out a way to get rid of you; you've seen them do that to other professors. You'll lose your reputation, your car, your house. Everyone will be laughing at you, mocking you, saying they always knew you weren't up to the job—that you were a fuckup.*

"A *fuckup*?" I ask, emphasizing the harshness of his words.

Armand inclines his head, a gesture hovering between assent and apology. "When I was a kid, I was always screwing things up. We used to vacation in Spain every summer. My older brother took me out one day to look for *girolles*—chanterelles. He was seven years older. We each had a basket. I was six, maybe seven. He showed me what to look for, and I said, 'Okay.' I thought I knew how to tell one kind of mushroom from another and separate out the look-alikes. But when we got back, I'd only collected two chanterelles; the rest were inedible; several were poisonous. I remember my brother shaking my basket upside down and saying, 'You're such a loser, you can't do anything right! What a fuckup! You're so ridiculous—look at you! What were you trying to do, kill us?'"

Armand didn't just hear about this mishap once. "I had to rehear it every time my brother told it to my mother, my father, my grandmother, his friends." Armand laughs. "Look, I definitely had attention issues as a kid. I was kind of a mess. But all my little screwups were used by my family to entertain other people, and not in a cute sitcom-like way. It was more like, 'Do you remember the time Armand . . . ha ha ha ha ha ha ha!' Whenever we had guests over, we'd have these long, long dinners, and my parents would ask me to play the piano. I was pretty good at the piano. But I'd get nervous and mess up, and my father would sigh and say to all his professor friends, 'He doesn't *listen*! He doesn't *try*. If he listened to his teacher, he'd be able to play that piece! You can't imagine the money I've spent!'" To this day, Armand can still hear everyone laughing at his father's "joke."

Often, Armand would end up clapping his hands over his ears so he couldn't hear anything more, yelling at his father, "Stop! Stop! Stop!" and bursting into tears before running to his room and slamming the door.

Armand's most painful memory is of his father teaching him math after dinner at the kitchen table. "My dad was a pretty well-known math professor. If I brought home a quiz with anything less than one hundred percent, he'd slam his fist on the table and say, 'Not good enough, Armand!' He'd make up dozens of drill sheets and keep me up until two in the morning. I wasn't allowed to go to bed until I did ten sets of ten problems perfectly. While I was working, he'd tell me, 'So-and-so's son is getting perfect scores in math! Don't you know how embarrassing it is for me that you don't try harder?'" Armand's mom was softer, but she was pretty checked out by then. She was older; he'd been a "surprise," and by the time he came along, she was "sipping wine with lunch and didn't stop until she fell asleep." But even she sometimes belittled him, once quite publicly when she showed up at a soccer game at his school. Watching from the sidelines, she called out, "Armand! Try harder!" When they were in the car driving home afterward, she said, "I'm so glad your father wasn't there; he'd be so disappointed."

It was around then, in high school, that Armand's friends stopped coming over. "My best friend in high school told me his mom said he couldn't come to my house anymore; she didn't think it was a 'good environment for kids.'" A few years later, when Armand and his high school girlfriend broke up, "my mom's first words were 'What did you *do?*' Then my dad started in: 'She was too good for you! Of course she didn't want to keep dating you! She saw how lazy you are!'"

When Armand left for college in the United States, his father's last words to him in the airport were "Don't mess up! Don't crack up, Armand!"

In college, Armand took several psychology classes. One day, a professor was diagramming a dysfunctional family on the board to explain how parental behavior and immaturity could affect a child's sense of self-worth. "I had this dizzying moment when I realized that the family he was describing was mine." The professor outlined how growing up with an immature parent—one whose ego is so large and needy they can't validate or acknowledge the reality of their child's emotional experience—could leave a child with insecure attachment.

Armand decided to see the school counselor, who referred him to an outside therapist. But Armand needed his parents to sign on for this; otherwise, how would he pay for it? He decided to ask his parents for their support when he went home for winter break. When he put the question before them, he used words that were thoughtful and devoid of blame: "I told my parents I was struggling with a lot of test anxiety, and a counselor had suggested that seeing an outside therapist in Boston might help me get to the root of it, which would help me academically. They'd given me a referral, and if I went twice a month, it would only cost a few hundred dollars." But this did not go over well. "My parents were seething.

My father said, 'Armand, you need to settle down. You're doing this so you have someone to blame other than yourself. It's your own doing! It's your fault you can't focus. You get nervous because you know you're lazy!' " Armand responded as calmly as he could, "Maybe we could *all* use help to improve our family dynamic and how we interact with one another." That enraged his father, who told him, "Armand! You cause all the strife in our family with your resentment and anger! *You* are the one with the problem! You need to get a grip on yourself or you're going to crack up!"

When he went back to college, Armand didn't see a therapist. He began to struggle even more. Unable to fall asleep at night, he overslept and started missing class. "When I did make it to class, instead of trying to catch up, I'd panic about how far behind I'd fallen and spend the whole time worrying how much trouble I'd be in once my parents found out I was failing."

A few weeks later, Armand was told by his academic dean that he needed to take a break from school and go home for the rest of that term. When he called his parents to tell them he was on academic leave, his father yelled over the transatlantic connection, "I always *knew* you'd crack up!"

Today, fifteen years later, instead of enjoying finally achieving tenure, Armand finds himself "walking into meetings hearing my dad's voice in the back of my head. It's like my father is hiding in the corner of every room."

Armand doesn't want that. Nor does he deserve it. He wants to spend his precious mental energy figuring out "a vision for our department in an era when the humanities are under fire." He wants to enjoy more moments of "clarity and ideation; those times when I can easily and clearly discern which ideas are worth keeping and building upon." Armand's voice grows stronger as he speaks about how such moments of unfettered inspiration feel. "I'm talking about those moments of knowing, really knowing inside of me, when I'm onto something. But I can't enter into the ideas that give my work meaning when I'm expending my energy on trying to shut off the fire hose of my internal lambasting."

I gave him some ideas about the practices I described in the preceding chapters, and he tried a few, with encouraging results. But his motivation to change became a lot stronger when, a few months later, he and his wife had their first child. "I'm a father now," Armand told me when I called to congratulate him and also to see how he was doing with the various practices. "I don't want to worry, while I raise my son, if I'm capable of being a good-enough dad, or flashing back to things my father did and said to me as a kid and overcorrecting, or, worse, finding I'm like my father because I don't know how else to be." From that time on, he began to really focus on what he needed to do to become the father he wanted to be—and the person.

At heart, Armand wants what I want, and what you probably want, too: "an infallible, portable utility belt to help me land in a place of sanctuary so that I can be with all that is good, all that is possible, in my life, in my relationships, and within me."

Perhaps because he's a professor, Armand has diagrammed his ruminations for me, and how he escapes them. He shows me the paper on which he's decoded his ruminations. It reads like the perfect student's—or, as in this case, professor's—homework, or better yet, the perfect crib sheet for what to do when we're enmeshed in our mind drama.

First, Armand uses MIST to capture the mental movies, intense emotions, and somatic sensations that most often arise for him after a triggering event, which he describes as follows:

Mental movies: Flashes of moments being berated by my father, mother, and brother, kitchen table, piano, nearly failing out of college.

Intense internal emotions: Shame, self-loathing, self-hatred, fear of being judged, loss of confidence, feeling paranoid everyone thinks I'm a loser, a fuckup.

Somatic sensations: Head hot like an inferno, constricted pressure on chest, heart pounding, gasping for sips of air, palms sweat.

Tie it all together: *Here's my old story of how I'm so ridiculous, a screwup/fuckup, which fills me with shame and turns my head into a hot, self-loathing inferno.*

For extra credit, Armand has added these reminders to his crib sheet:

Remind Myself:

1. This starts happening in my default mode network before I'm consciously aware of it. If I don't intervene, my default mode will keep playing these stories on an infinite loop like the spinning beach ball of death on my computer.
2. Armand, this is a signal fire from your past, calling for your attention, your self-compassion!
3. You didn't sign up for this, Armand! You didn't agree to sign on to these derogatory self-beliefs when you were a child! You don't have to now! You don't have to let this story dog you anymore.
4. How do you want to take care of yourself right now? What will help you feel safe? How can you offer yourself the kind of compassion you didn't get as a kid?

Armand has also created a set of reminders as to his favorite practices to help him move toward a greater feeling of clarity, safety, and possibility:

Ballistic interrupters: "I'm not expending my precious energy on this. I'm proud of myself for doing this work so I can be a better parent and a happier person. I'm moving past my old stories."

Body-state breakers (when with others): Physiological sighing.

Body-state breakers (when alone): Go for a run or lift weights, cold shower for three minutes, play music whole time, try shaking it out. Dance to music with my son in my arms.

Cultivate opposite feeling: Flash Technique while watching the look on my son's face as he sleeps. Drawing his face. Remembering my fear can be my friend.

I tell Armand I'm bowled over by his self-awareness and effort. "When you first told me what you were writing about," he said in response, "I was afraid these practices might further immerse me into my worst thoughts. But then I saw the countervailing argument. Excavating where these thoughts come from and why they keep trying to get my attention helps me see them in a new light. And I'm able to respond to them in a way that helps me process that pain. By seeing what they're trying to tell me, and being vulnerable with myself in this way, my brain is no longer so obsessed with trying to replay my past stories. I'm starting to feel freed from their hold. And that makes me feel I can maybe even accomplish some of the things I hope to do in my field. I'm more hopeful. Some days, I'm even excited about the future." (One note here: If it seems Armand is a quick study, he is. In full disclosure, he is now in therapy, which no doubt helps him explain his experiences so succinctly. On that note, as I've said before, doing this work with a therapist to help you along is a fantastic way to enhance your healing.)

Armand's journey is marvelously illustrative of all the mind hacks and work I've outlined thus far. But his story is also a great example of what's possible: By doing this work, he has begun to open the door to that wider expanse of ideation and creativity that's waiting for all of us when we exit our mind drama. He has figured out a way to give more oxygen to his authentic, creative force.

In this, I move from being Armand's guide to being his student. I'll let Armand tell you how he came to have a deeper connection to the freewheeling muse within him.

"When I was a child and was being yelled at, I'd focus on an object in the room: a person's nose, a belt buckle, the glossy tip of a shoelace, a pair of glasses someone had left on the table. I'd play this game in my head where I'd zoom in on that object and observe every detail, almost as if I were able to make myself very small and walk around it and see it up close. It was soothing and calming. In therapy, I learned that this was a way of dissociating, escaping a painful situation. But I didn't know that when I was a kid. All I knew was that observing things in minute detail somehow comforted me, and it also led me to start looking closely at faces and doodling portraits of them. I'd draw the faces of friends, teachers, classmates, sometimes on my homework. My friends got a kick out of it. My teachers actually didn't mind. One teacher I drew wrote in a margin once, 'Nice likeness!' But my father thought it was a waste of time. It meant I wasn't paying attention in class. If he caught me drawing, he'd rip it up. So I stopped."

Recently, Armand picked up drawing again—not stick figures, not doodles, but real portraits. "I have always had this interest in people's facial features. Everyone's face is so unique. At conferences, if I'm in a room with a lot of people and no one is going to notice, I'll draw people's expressions. Maybe, because I'm a little bit neurodivergent, it's my way of trying to understand people better. What they feel. Who they are."

Lately, Armand began drawing his newborn son, "his tiny fingers, his small, perfect face. I wanted to capture him as he's changing; he's changing so fast!" Today, Armand carries a small sketch pad with him wherever he goes. "When my mind is playing tricks on me and my dad's voice is blaring inside, and I start to get that hot, shameful, *'Armand, you're such a fuckup' feeling in my head*—I pick up my sketch pad." Armand draws the most interesting face he sees or remembers having seen. It preempts "all the negative stuff" and gives him an opportunity to direct his mental energy to something creative and fulfilling. "Not only have I stopped the old story that was sucking me in, but suddenly, I'm thinking more expansively.

About everything. My relationships. My work. It's as if that one, small creative act cross-pollinates and makes everything in my mind fertile ground for growth."

Armand feels he's "relating to the world on a new level. I'm more connected in my relationships. It's helping me feel more attached to my son. I always worried if I had a son, I wouldn't be able to connect with him because of that muscle memory I have that intimacy brings with it a total break of trust, which brought me tremendous pain as a kid. I worried I'd be so driven by fear I wouldn't be able to feel this . . . this awe I have that someone so beautiful and innocent is here. The possibility of loss would have kept me from knowing him."

Allowing himself license to be creative has opened Armand up in other ways: "The more I draw people's faces, the more compassion I feel for all of us. I see so much suffering and fatigue and worry in people's eyes and expressions. They, too, have wounds that have left them feeling alone, and separate, and apart. In this way, we're all the same. And yet at the same time, I see how each face, each person, is so beautiful and full of gifts in their own way. If we can see this in each other, we can connect."

Accompanying Yourself to the Past

This exploration of his creative capability has increased Armand's capacity to turn toward his own pain, and helped make his understanding of how much weight he's been carrying from his childhood really concrete. One day, as he was doodling, Armand found himself drawing his five-year-old self—who was drawing in the dirt with a stick. And then he found himself having a daydream in which he went over and crouched down and talked to that little kid, who seemed to be crying, his dirty face streaked with tears. Armand gently wiped off his kid self's face and told him, "Hey, hey, it's going to be okay—we're going to be okay." Then his kid self showed Armand what he was drawing in the dirt—he was trying to draw a beetle he'd been watching. He told Armand, through his tears, that his father had looked at his drawing and laughed at him when he told him it was of a beetle. Armand kept telling his kid self, "It's really going to be okay, little guy. I'm here now," all the while thinking, *Hey, I have to honor this kid's experience, by doing what I need to do now to heal, so I can be the father I want to be to my son... and be who I want to be in this life I get to live.*

There are many ways of putting ourselves back into our minds as a child, and Armand found his way intuitively to it through drawing. After Armand told me, with tears in his own eyes, about this powerful experience, I decided to ask neuropsychiatrist Ruth Lanius about why accompanying ourselves to the past in this way can help foster our healing. (Bridging between our adult and child selves is a premise many therapeutic practices draw upon to help us relieve the burdened parts of ourselves.)

Lanius explains there is a good, neuroscience-based reason why these approaches work: We are using what we know of the default mode network to our advantage. "Our trauma memories are not time-stamped," she explains. "We can go back and revisit that time, those events, those years, when we were not received or accepted, when our pain was neglected, and when our default mode network wired up in response to those messages—and help ourselves to process and relieve that pain now."

When you have a history of early adversity, Lanius says, the front hub of your default mode network (the dorsal medial prefrontal cortex), which roots you in the present, and the back hub (the posterior cingulate cortex), which keeps you reliving old experiences, stop talking to each other. When this happens, you keep reexperiencing the old experiences without a time stamp. Something might be a memory, but it feels like it's still happening to you now.

You can use words to strengthen the connection between these two hubs. When you mentally time travel and use the language of your calmer, loving, present adult self to comfort and validate your younger, past self, "you allow your present-centeredness to filter into the part of your default mode network that's still caught in the past. You become a mental time traveler who can voluntarily travel back into the past to help your younger self heal, versus being involuntarily ripped back into the past. You bring your past and your present selves together."

The French philosopher Simone Weil said that "attention, taken to its highest degree, is the same thing as prayer." What I hear and see in Armand is something like this: an ignited sense of attention that expands, fueled by its own velocity, into awe. Armand is experiencing the sensation of being molecularly awake. All this because he has, by accessing his creative imagination, successfully brought his child self and his adult self together, across time—right in the default mode network of his mind.

Channeling Your Rumination for Creativity and Growth

Rumination clearly lies at the heart of much that is ugly and destructive, but also so much that is beautiful. Yet the more liberating, generative aspect of rumination has mainly gone unexplored in the popular press, even as it has recently become a topic of interest to researchers who view it as the doorway into an active inner space where new ideas and creativity thrive.

Psychologist Mihaly Csikszentmihalyi, author of the books *Flow* and *Creativity*, writes about how creativity offers us "a central source of meaning in our lives," which delivers us into those moments that make life worth living. When we are immersed in creativity, we live more fully.

There is a good reason why the word *muse* is found in *Merriam-Webster*'s description of rumination and is also used to describe the deepest source of our creative inspiration. In 1822, Marie-Henri Beyle, better known as the novelist Stendhal, wrote *On Love*, in which love itself is described as an act of the imagination. Stendhal was inspired by his ruminations over why we love, how we love, when love starts to brew, and how it changes us over time. He couldn't stop musing over and analyzing these questions. *On Love* is the timeless result. Many creatives and thought leaders say their biggest breakthroughs arose during hours when they fell deep into the good rabbit hole of an open, ruminating attention, lost in a kind of mind-wandering that stimulated ingenuity and imagination. "I believe in rumination and lose half the beauty of all things when I am deprived of the time to ruminate," writer Anaïs Nin wrote. Actor Daniel Day-Lewis once said he spends "many months in apparently listless rumination out of which I hope something will emerge." (Clearly, something does.)

Few among us will ever be the next Stendhal or Nin or Day-Lewis. That's not the goal. This is: the ability to channel your ruminations so that they become the source of your capacity for action, change, and growth. This is why you don't want to view your growing awareness of how your mind drama can derail you as simply an impetus to shut down that overthinking. Instead, you want to reroute it, to discover what awaits you when you shift out of the dark side of that state and allow your brain to begin humming with ideas and images that inspire you.

I wonder if you have known this feeling, too. When you begin—like Armand—to feel that interior sense of play, awe, and flow, it's not just your mind but your physiology that shifts. Levels of stress hormones go down, fast, as does your heart rate. You calm your nervous system. Increased levels of good hormones that promote compassion, love, trust, and bonding, like oxytocin, are released. In rare instances, you might even feel that tingling sensation that accompanies a big aha moment, an epiphany, the excitement of a new awareness or idea.

Cognitive psychologist Scott Barry Kaufman, director of the Center for Human Potential, has emerged as a leading voice in rethinking the role of the default mode network, arguing that it can also be a core driver of our highest creative thinking. He's challenging the conventional wisdom, arguing that this area of the brain is crucial for unlocking the kind of imaginative cognition that propels innovation—a perspective that is gaining traction in neuroscience circles. In researching what human imagination and inspiration look like in the brain, Kaufman and his colleagues have shown that we draw upon our default mode network not just for "our self-narratives" or to "access deeply personal episodic memories from our past" but for our creative thinking. This includes "daydreaming, planning for the future, the mental visualization of our future self," and "the awe and openness that arise from new experiences." But here's the catch: To play this positive, adaptive role, and shift out of its negative, overactive, ruminative state, the default mode network has to fully interface with the wider brain, including areas responsible for higher thinking, decision-making, and wise choices. "It's the integration" of these areas "that matters."

Just as it would be misguided to view rumination as wholly undesirable, it would be shortsighted to view the default mode network as solely "the villain, the source of our suffering," Kaufman rightly argues. When we coax the default mode network to synchronize with our whole brain, it becomes the "hero, not the villain." Using brain scans, Kaufman has shown how true this is. In a recent study, he compared two groups. The first group of twenty individuals was comprised of what Kaufman terms "eminent thinkers" and "creators from diverse fields of expertise" who had demonstrated high levels of "lifetime creative achievement." The second group, the control group, was comprised of sixteen people of similar ages and educational backgrounds as the eminent thinkers. These participants were extremely "smart" but hadn't reached similar levels of lifetime achievement in their creative fields. Both groups were given creative tasks to complete while undergoing fMRI scans. Big differences emerged: The default mode networks of the eminent thinkers interacted with networks "across the brain" both when they were engaged in tasks and when they were at rest, in a way the "smart" group's did not.

Similarly, researchers at the University of North Carolina at Greensboro recently found via fMRI scans that our "ability to generate creative ideas" requires "increased functional creativity" between the default mode network and the prefrontal cortex—that is, between the area that is the source of our mind-wandering, and the area that is responsible for our executive function. Whole-brain neural integration really matters. Life is full of challenges that require the motherboards across our brains to light up and interface. This is true across every domain of our lives, whether it's troubleshooting a new home security system, problem-solving during a family crisis, honing our best ideas for a high-stakes meeting, or writing a poem or a symphony—all of which require creativity.

Two-time Oscar winner Emma Stone hasn't had her brain scanned by Kaufman, but the way she thinks about the role rumination has played in her life sounds very similar to what he describes. In a conversation with *Fresh Air* host Terry Gross, Stone recounted how learning to harness the fear-based stories in her head has made her a better actress. She also talked about how being an actress, and the creativity and passion required, have helped her learn how to manage worried thought spirals.

Even as a teen, Stone struggled with worrisome what-ifs about the future, she explained to Gross. She worried about what if their house caught on fire or what if something bad happened to her mother. Even now, she confided, she too often gets caught up in "either future tripping or past tripping." Over time, however, she has taught herself to utilize rumination as a force for creativity, by realizing that "intuition and anxiety" about the future come out of the same place, "that same spot." The trick, for her, lies in learning to distinguish between the "racing" heart and fiery feeling that herald her fear-based ruminations, and the interior "calm, like a knowing and a warmth," that fills her in creative moments. In the former, she feels terrified and overwhelmed; in the latter, she feels safe and called to do something bigger. We certainly see something very ambitious—and meaningful—in

Poor Things, the 2023 film for which Stone won the Oscar for best actress. One of the best things about being able to exit her fear-based ruminations and open herself to the upside of rumination, Stone told Gross, is finding the safety she needs inside her body to do something creative in a high-stakes moment—of which there were an extraordinary number in *Poor Things.*

I know that many of my own ruminations can seem to bring forth the same feelings of both fear and joy that Stone talks about, which open me up to something larger than myself. I think back to a harrowing chapter in my life: my late thirties and early forties, when my children were small, and I was repeatedly paralyzed by a rare neurological disorder. The fear was primal, sharpened by the memory of losing my father when I was young. I was terrified of leaving my children in the same way. The physical pain was relentless, stretching on for months. Even now, my mind gets trapped in memories of how frightened my children were, how frightened I was. I get caught in thought circles about the toll those years took, especially on my youngest, who still carries a shadow of those bewildering days.

But if I can stop and reorient my ruminations into something more expansive, a different kind of feeling arises. I find myself viewing the story of our family not just as a series of hardships but as a tapestry woven with resilience, a quiet grace. I gain perspective, even a little awe, over the things we have endured together. Yes, there have been unimaginable heartbreaks—as there are in any family—but also a quiet tenderness that has threaded its way through even our darkest moments. I marvel at that, within us all, which propels us on through fear and loss, to find each other on the other side. And once I can pull back to that place of perspective, I feel a sense of wonder at how any of us are able to survive experiences that can, for swaths of time, leave us hollowed out by fear and suffering—and how we find our way back again.

Something larger and more embracing then calls to me: a desire to help others facing their challenges—something I hope my books enable me to do, if only in some small way. When I can stop experiencing my churning, ruminating thoughts and shift into this more sweeping, self-aware, and connected state, I feel the whisper of something bigger: a clarity of purpose, a vibrant imagination that sometimes delivers me into a sense of certainty about what to do or say, or how to be that better parent, partner, or friend (including a better friend to myself), or what I want to convey in whatever book or article or talk I'm creating at that moment. In high-flow moments—which arise most often in my personal, private writing—I feel my whole being pour itself into the effort, until it feels like no effort at all. In some deep, internal place, I feel more open and alive, brimming over with a melting tenderness toward everything and everyone.

The new science on rumination tells us that we have within ourselves the power to not only extricate ourselves from the dark side of ruminating and set out on a very different, purposeful path but to enter the upside of rumination, and almost at will.

When we are no longer so seduced by our mind drama, we can regain and redirect our ill-spent mental energy. Given that, according to the research, we spend four-plus hours a day caught up in mind drama, that's a very large bonus of time. And like Armand, we can then use that time to give breath to our creative thinking and endeavors.

How can we awaken these deeper layers of creative energy, inventiveness, and imagination? This requires us to dig a bit deeper. But I'm confident that everything this requires is well within our reach—and we might even discover the process to be genuinely, joyfully transformative.

FOURTEEN

What Does It Look Like When We Get Out of Our Own Way?

HOW DO YOU open up to the power of healthy mind-wandering and creative ideation, and reclaim your ill-spent mental energy in ways that fulfill you? Thanks to new advances in neuroimaging, the science on how to tap into the upside of rumination is becoming robust. One of the best ways to get there is by enhancing your brain's receptivity to the muse that's already within you. Below, you'll discover a set of strategies inspired by new research on the default mode network, offering fresh ways to spark creativity and fuel your Inner Muse.

Allow Your Mind to Race Free

We can't enter that state in which we feel our Inner Muse move with us and through us unless we release our minds and let go of our desire to control and manage our thoughts. Scott Barry Kaufman's explorations of the positive aspects of mind-wandering build on work that psychologist Jerome L. Singer wrote about in his research on constructive daydreaming sixty years ago. Kaufman, like Singer, argues that choosing to disengage from external tasks and decouple our attention from what's going on around us "to pursue an internal stream of thought" is "central to the task of meaning making, of developing and maintaining an understanding of oneself in the world."

While much of our mind-wandering happens beneath our awareness, we can actively choose to allow our minds to roam free. Letting your daydreams flow, while gently nudging them toward whatever creative challenge lies at hand, can help brain networks that don't usually cooperate with one another form stronger connections.

Alison Gopnik, a UC Berkeley philosopher, has, like Scott Barry Kaufman, found that when we ruminate in a reflective, open way, it "becomes a positive feature of cognition. Letting our thoughts drift can help us solve problems. A free association thought process that randomly generates memories and imaginative experiences leads us to new ideas and insights." Gopnik likens this open, creative mental state to having a "lantern-like consciousness," which differs from the way we usually go through life, "shining a spotlight" on our problems, and seeing little else. In this lantern-like light, we not only see possible solutions to problems that have been bedeviling us, we land on that which is most useful and true. (Or as Emma Stone put it in her conversation with Terry Gross on *Fresh Air*, you feel a "kind of deep knowing" within you to go a certain way.)

You can begin to shed that light more brightly by giving your Inner Muse permission to enter a free-floating state of uncensored thought. Some of the ideas bubbling up from the depths will prove to be terrible, but some of them may be very good indeed. Let your mind wander now. You can edit later.

Here, it might help to think of your brain as having two systems:

- System 1 is your creative supplier; it generates that stream of new ideas that seem to emanate from nowhere. As you practice and explore, you invite yourself to make mistakes, give yourself permission to create junk, things you will later throw away.

- System 2 is a slower, more deliberate, more conscious state of creativity, in which you consider those spontaneous ideas you've generated, reviewing what you've created with objectivity, deciding what to build upon while discarding the rest. "Creativity is a wild mind and a disciplined eye," writer Dorothy Parker once reportedly said. Both are required.

This two-step process of sequentially utilizing both your "inner supplier" and your "inner critic" aligns with the neuroscience on creativity. First, your default mode network runs free with daydreaming and introspection as you try new ways to go at something. Then, those ideas are sifted and sorted through under the supervision of your executive control network. You bring in your cooler, more critical eye, as needed, to see what is working best and build from there.

So write haiku, design crossword puzzles, paint watercolors, sink your hands into clay and make things, shoot short films with your smartphone, build a bird box or simple piece of furniture, experiment with nature photography, become a bird-watcher, learn more about an era of art that fills you with awe and visit museums so you can stand in front of those works with your sketchbook in hand, take your love of cooking to the next level, pick up the recorder you stopped playing in the fifth grade. Almost anything that entices and calls to you can fit into this category.

What you're going for here is to experience one of life's greatest pleasures—the joy that comes when you and your Inner Muse become part of a larger, magical, creative moment in which time stops and the workings of your imagination become largely automatic and unconscious. Brian Eno, the inventor of generative music, urges us to choose "not to be imprisoned by our smartness" but to instead celebrate our freedom to enter the creative state he calls "idiot glee."

Keep Doing It—Whatever "It" Is

People often think of creativity as a bolt of sudden inspiration, and there are moments when those do happen; but the more patiently and consistently you give yourself over to developing a skill, the more frequently such moments will occur. Putting time and practice into your creative pursuit really pays off. This is true partly because with more practice, you will feel confident enough to release control and let go, which allows your brain networks to hum in harmony with little or no conscious supervision. Your brain starts to create on "autopilot" without interference. It's not unlike physical fitness. The more you work your creative muscles, the stronger they get. Indeed, John Kounios, a psychologist at Drexel University who studies creativity, has shown this on brain scans. In one study using neuroimaging to look at the brains of jazz musicians as they were playing, Kounios found that the more experience the musicians had, the easier access they had to the effortless attention that allowed them to enter a creative flow state.

Kounios's findings make sense to Virginia, who is still growing as an artist. "The more I paint, the more I see things I couldn't see before; and the more aware I then become of what I want and need to paint, where to focus my eye, what to do with my paintbrush. It's not conscious. While I'm painting, I'm not aware of anything except the work in front of me. There is no past, no future, only now and what is happening on the canvas. And that is a very powerful feeling. I think it is the only way to get into that playful state of creativity that is essential for art. You make work without fear, because you are so lost in the moment, you don't care how it turns out. Fear of being rejected is the biggest issue for artists. It's in an environment where fear is totally unnecessary that art happens. I'm on the path toward becoming the artist I'm capable of being by finding ways to tamp down the fear I've always felt—which is just another word for *rumination.*"

Later, Virginia can return to the work and think about what it might need to make it better. "You have to be able to tell the critic to go away, or you won't be able to make the thing. Once you've made it, you can invite the inner critic to come back and ask it, 'Is this right? What part of this works?' "

Kounios's work, and Virginia's experience, recall John Lennon's words, "If you start a song, write it through to the end in that sitting. Don't be concerned if some of the parts are not yet all they can be. Get through a rough draft." You can always edit later.

Virginia likens this state of creation without fear to what children do. "You know how when kids are playing and they're doing dopey little things without any awareness that anyone is watching, they're singing to themselves, they're hopping around on one foot, they're throwing themselves into their finger painting? They're just lost in the joy of what they're doing." That is creativity at work, and it's a lesson she has had to relearn. "Little kids are not busy critiquing their own play. And artists can't critique their work as they make it." As Virginia's Inner Muse becomes ever-more confident, "negative comments don't matter as much anymore. I am finally able to take what I need and let the rest go. Sure, that little voice—'You suck'—is still there, but it's whispering now and barely heard, because I no longer care about other people's judgments. I'm just not interested in that anymore."

Recently, Virginia channeled this newly freed energy into building a new studio. She was frustrated by how often family members kept walking in on her when she picked up her paintbrush. "I crave silence, space, time, without anyone coming into my studio to ask me if I'm going to walk the dog or what's for dinner. But my family sees me as constantly interruptible. Rather than wait for them to change, I realized that if I wanted to have the mental silence I crave, I would have to change the situation." And Virginia did. She built a small art studio in their backyard, about twice the size of a shed, with electricity, running water, and large windows. "I had to honor that voice inside that told me I deserved to create an environment in which I was free to express myself."

After talking to Virginia, I went to visit her new studio.

The northern light streaming in through the large back window is steady and inviting. Paintings, smocks, tubes of paint, lie everywhere in happy, ordered chaos. The studio door opens onto her garden, which gives her utter privacy. But what stands out most, as I look around, is how Virginia has changed. Maybe it's the scattered paintbrushes, the late-afternoon light, or the way her copper hair, freed from its chignon, falls in easy waves. But there's something new in her presence—she's steady, unguarded—her gaze more direct, her body relaxed and quietly assured, seeming to announce that she's deep in her element. "No one comes in. No one disturbs me until I come out of my studio. I'm the keeper of my own time. And that allows my brain to generate more ideas, without fear of whether they are good or bad." Virginia would make another Virginia—Virginia Woolf—proud: She's created a room of her own, tucked away from the demands that so often hold women back from their artistic expression.

Recently, a gallery known for its watercolor artists asked to represent Virginia's work, and they've sold quite a few. "I forget who said, 'Don't die with your music still inside you,'" she tells me. "But that's how I feel. I don't want to die with my song—the things I see and feel—still locked inside me. Will I regret spending some of our retirement money to build my studio? I don't think so. I know when I retire, I'll lean more into my art, and I'll be eternally grateful to my younger self that she made this investment on behalf of my future self."

But there is, Virginia tells me, a bigger payoff to leaving her ruminations behind her. "It allows me to love myself better, and more, and in doing so I'm more able to love the people around me and convey that love to them. And that is the most powerful thing of all."

Virginia is what it looks like when we get out of our own way.

This idea that there are payoffs beyond the immediate work is one that Armand believes in, too. Unlike Virginia, Armand isn't focused on becoming an artist. But when he's sketching, "I don't just capture ideas that help me with how to draw a nose, or someone's hair, or capture the light," Armand tells me. "I have mini insights that offer solutions to things worrying me in other areas of my life. It's like the answers come toward me. I start to see how I might talk to one of my grad students who is struggling, or what I want to say to my wife about a conversation we had."

This is the power of the creative mind, when we allow it to work on our behalf. It's as if ideas are asking us to dance with them, and we have only to accept their invitation.

Play!

Monotony can rob your brain of your creativity and sense of wonder. One of NASA's concerns in sending humans to live on Mars for extended periods of time is that the monotony of life on the barren planet might interfere with human ingenuity in ways that could be harmful to the space mission. Closer to home, in one study by researchers at McGill University, when students were put in cubicles for long periods, it led to "a change of attitude": They ruminated more about their studies and personal woes. Eventually, they lost their ability to focus.

Here's the takeaway: Don't be afraid to try new things. Open up your world just a little more. Step out of your comfort zone. Do hard things. Learn, explore, try, fail, get lost along the way, and find yourself on an unfamiliar path. At the Torrance Center for Creativity at the University of Georgia, psychologist Anna Abraham has found that "across different age groups, the best predictor of creativity is openness to new experiences." That "curiosity that draws you toward learning new things and experiencing the world in new ways." And yes—you know this science by now—your openness to experience emanates from a default mode network that is humming in connection with the networks in the rest of the brain.

Creativity is the ability to "strike out in new directions"

and create new things or do old things in new ways, developmental psychologist Howard Gardner wrote. But this process is not passive. You have to seek out ideas, people, places, and things that inspire you.

Maria Popova, author of the blog *The Marginalian* and the book *Figuring*, once told a reporter from *Mother Jones* that to move from rumination ("I have bad days. Sometimes I have a *lot* of bad days. . . . I think most people fall into a bad mood because they're able to ruminate on whatever the problem at hand is, and that makes it worse") to a "stimulating and absorbing" mind-wandering, she "consumes 12 to 15 books a week." She's looking for hidden gems, "stuff that a little bit, in a tiny way changes how you see something about the world." We all carry a lot of "knowledge and insight and inspiration," she said, and "over time, these Lego bricks . . . build this enormous, incredible castle." It seems to me that Popova's creative mind-wandering is the culmination of all these gems she's collected, or, as she puts it, it arises from all "these interesting pieces of stuff that we carry and accumulate over the course of our lives," which she then is able to "recombine into new things" in a way that is wholly and uniquely her own.

We may not have a mind that can make words sing like Popova's, but we can all make a concerted effort to outfit our lives with activities and people we find enriching. Vary your daily walk, take day trips, meet your friends at museums or parks instead of talking on the phone or going to the same corner restaurant, talk to strangers at the dog run, make new friends.

Recently, I heard an anecdote from a friend, which, to me, exemplified this courage to try new things. Her neighbor, eighty-one, took up the cello last year. Everyone assumed it would be a passing fancy, because what could possibly come of trying to learn such a difficult instrument at such an advanced age when he didn't even know how to read music when he began? And yet, after a year of practice and dedication, his music teacher suggested he join an amateur quartet. He did, and the joy he now takes in it is palpable, written "across his face," my friend reports. "His eyes light up with pleasure when he talks about it, his words overflow with excitement." At a time when he had been somewhat at loose ends, retired and not quite knowing what to do with himself, he has found a sense of passion, purpose, and agency as he ages.

Picasso said, "It takes me a long time to be young." It takes a long time for all of us, sometimes a lifetime, to return to that state of play, wonder, and astonishment that we so often leave behind in childhood, only to miss it more with every passing year.

Mix It Up!

After encouraging you to dive deep into your passions, it might sound contradictory to warn that studies show that if you focus your attention too narrowly, it can hinder ingenuity. Mihaly Csikszentmihalyi argues that we are most likely to find what sparks that sense of aha and wonder in us when we marry disparate disciplines: "The most creative individuals are those who are able to connect disparate domains, to see relationships where others see none." One of my favorite writers, when I was a child, was Madeleine L'Engle, author of the beloved children's classic *A Wrinkle in Time.* L'Engle was inspired by molecular biology in writing her stories—and that is part of what makes her tales both magical and believable.

I find this idea very helpful—and reconfirming. It makes me think how my entire career (which I do find very creative and engaging; I am always learning something new) is built on the desire to draw from ideas in many different fields. When I was a young undergrad at Duke University, many decades ago, I struggled to fit in all the classes that interested me on top of my basic requirements. Public policy, English literature, poetry, women's studies, and creative writing / journalism—I wanted to study all of it. One day, I met with my academic dean to talk about my dilemma. I told her these were all areas I wanted to pursue, and combine, perhaps in journalism or some other form of writing. Or maybe teaching. I didn't know. I explained to her that I'd grown up with a newspaper editor father who'd been devoted to creating a better, fairer world and active in shaping public policy and discourse. On my mother's side, I'd grown up surrounded by scientists. But I also wanted to do something to help women, especially young women, who'd experienced trauma and loss. I'd just finished a photojournalism project, in which I'd followed a group of girls living in a halfway house, who had shared with me their stories of growing up in troubled homes. My life changed when, after listening to me ramble, she (thank you, Dean Wittig, wherever you are) said, long before interdisciplinary majors were an option, "Why don't we create an interdisciplinary major around all these things?" I can still recall the elation I felt as I thanked her and flew out of her office, brimming with excitement, yes, but something more, that feeling of "I can." The answer had been so simple. I didn't have to give up anything I loved; I could make space for all of it.

My friend Jasmine, who is an architect by trade, manages (like I do) a serious autoimmune condition, which can, when symptoms flare, trigger great rumination. Recently, Jasmine took a course at her local college to become a master gardener in her state of North Carolina. She's been able to marry her "love of design with gardening." She recently designed a labyrinth for a local park, which she crafted, in mosaic, from pieces of smoothed glass taken from broken bottles that once littered the park. "When I'm in the zone of creativity, self-consciousness and time disappear. I'm no longer in my stories of what's going to happen at the next appointment with my rheumatologist, or if I'm doing the right things to prevent progression of my disease, I'm just immersed in being here, right where I am."

Ada is doing something similar. She loves being a set designer—every aspect of it—scene design, production design, lighting design, "whatever helps with visual storytelling." But she also loves fashion and costume design—which are not her specialty. On a September morning when we meet up again, she wears simple blue leather slip-on sandals—her usual heels and vibrant red nail polish are gone, as if she's set aside some old vigilance. I notice, too, a new brightness in her face that speaks not of fretfulness but of having been in the sun, of laughter and unhurried afternoons. Ada seems more present to the world, more a companion to her own life than before. The change is not loud, but it is unmistakable. When I ask Ada about this vibe shift, she explains it thus: They have just returned—she, Carl, and their daughter—from their first vacation in six years. They wanted time to solidify their gains "in how we're communicating. And it was the best vacation we've ever had, not because we were in a beautiful place but because of how we were able to talk together so openly as a family."

It was important to Ada to take that time together before beginning a new venture that had her brimming with excitement. "I've always been a little jealous of the costume designers on set." While not a fashion hound per se, Ada loves to stitch and sew with her sewing machine, and she revels in "texture, textiles, color, and fabric. Bringing them together in just the right way can set the stage for a character, tell you who they are, and help an actor become that person." There is a lyric lift, a vitality, in Ada's voice, as she tells me about her plans. So, she continues, she has decided to go back to school part-time and get another master of arts degree in costume design.

Like Virginia, Ada's awakening is multifaceted. The work she's been doing, to step out of her mind drama, has helped her see how "I've been keeping myself small." As Ada has become clearer about who she is and who she wants to be, the "old stories that used to limit me have stopped haunting me. I guess at some point by doing this work, I started emotionally processing them without being aware I was doing so." Ada doesn't want to stay "hidden away in my little niche, working under difficult people, on their schedule, saying yes to all their whims." In a few years, with her added degree, she plans to "put together my own team, open my own company, and offer all aspects of set and film design, including costume design. I'll manage and oversee my own shop. That's the dream."

I'm curious how Ada's work has continued to affect her mother-daughter relationships. And here, too, more moments of magic have unfolded. "I can see now how much it must have hurt my mom when I just stopped talking to her when I was a teenager. I moved out when I was so young and never really came home again. When I was in college, I barely returned her phone calls, because just the thought of hearing her voice on the dorm phone put me into a panic. And yet she never stopped trying, no matter how many times I pushed her away. That had to be hard for her. Later, when I was older and had Allie, my mom kept calling, telling me she loved me, that she knew I would be a good mother, and she tried to set up visits even though it meant she had to fly all the way across the country. I always tried to find some excuse for her not to come. I regret how often I did that now."

Now that Ada has been able to step back and see how this pattern became echoed in her relationship with her daughter, she's gaining a "sixty-thousand-foot perspective. I see now, how in wanting to be close to Allie in a way I wasn't with my mom, I let my sense of myself as a mother be defined by how Allie behaved toward me. In the process, I missed something crucial: I didn't do the internal work on myself, first, so that I could give Allie the gift of being able to separate from me and be upset with me without my taking it personally. I resented her for not wanting me more in her life, and in that way, I became the very thing I didn't want to be—like my mom. That helps me to forgive my mom, to see myself in her, and her in me. I am not sure I can call it forgiveness for the *things* she said and did, but I definitely feel compassion. And that is new—a huge step up the ladder of emotions." Several times recently, Ada has picked up the phone and called her mom just to chat, not to talk about anything big. And their conversations are going "better than I would have thought. Recently, I told her about my plans to go back to school and set up my own company, and we ended up laughing about how when I was little, I'd make my own set designs and costumes and put on plays for my parents. I felt seen by her."

As for her relationship with Allie, "I've let go of that old fear that I'm not a good mom or that I'm being rejected by my own child." The relief in Ada's voice as she says this is palpable. This year, Ada's family and her mom are all getting together for Thanksgiving.

As I listen to Ada, I think, *This is what it looks like when a multigenerational wound begins to knit itself back together.*

Have Fun

Rick Rubin, author of *The Creative Act: A Way of Being* and a Grammy Award–winning music producer and record executive who has worked with many of the leading musicians of our time, says in his book that the most important thing you can do to foster your creativity and imagination is to give yourself permission to try something new, and see what emerges, without setting a goal. "Having a goal—that's not going to help you get there," he cautions. "It's more like, start finger painting and see what happens." If you want to play the piano, play the piano for five or ten minutes a day and simply tell yourself, "I'm gonna have fun." That might be a really nice gift to yourself. A pursuit for its own reward.

If you're not sure where to begin, think back to what filled you with glee—that uncomplicated state of wonder and joy—when you were a child. What made time fade away and brought you a greater sense of freedom, connectedness, and aliveness? When you lost track of everything around you, what were you doing? Did you love solving puzzles? Making jewelry? Reading mysteries? Did you love practicing magic? Building things? How can you spend time playing with that to which you have always felt drawn, in your adult life? Maybe you want to write cozy mysteries that you share with a circle of friends; wow your kids with magic card tricks; try your hand at building a shed in the backyard; learn cake decorating or flower arranging; or get a 3D printer and design things.

Armand has certainly done this with his drawing. He'd loved it as a child before his father destroyed his joy in it with his criticism. But now that he's doing it again, he's opened himself to a sense of "childlike seeing, and playfulness, that makes me feel so much more confident as a father. I never imagined I'd be that father who could get down on the floor and play with my child and enjoy it, or carry them around on my shoulders and point out birds in the trees, but I'm doing all those things. The more I allow myself to play, the more I feel drawn to play." (This brings to mind another piece of Rick Rubin's advice: "We're not playing to win, we're playing to play.")

This tenderness toward his young son has enlarged his tenderness toward himself. As Armand describes this interior shift, the old weight that once seemed to press down on him is gone, replaced by a quiet buoyancy. His hands move freely in front of him as if he is sketching the details of his life in the air before him, his gestures unhurried, emerging from a place of ease. He no longer seems to be always measuring, always weighing, always wondering: *Is this enough? Am I enough?* "I still have moments when I'm afraid, I'm worried I'm going to fuck up, get yelled at, be humiliated," he confides. "But then I tell myself I didn't have control over what happened to me. I can't go back and change what happened or turn back time to protect the little kid I was. But I can go back to be with him and acknowledge what happened to him. I can show little Armand, by my actions today, that I see him. I can comfort him and tell him, 'There was never anything wrong with you,' and reassure him, 'I will always protect you.' Because I feel him. He is still alive in me. And I carry him inside me with love, just as I carry my own child in my arms with love."

Sam grew up finding solace in hiking under a wide-open sky, coupled with a love of big sticks. Yes, sticks. Beautiful sticks. As a child, when he was really upset by something his dad had said to him, he'd head out on the wooded paths near his home.

"I'd take off down the trail, and just being in the woods, surrounded by trees, made whatever my dad had said to me less crushing. If I saw a big, beautiful stick, I'd pick it up and carry it like a staff, like Gandalf in *The Lord of the Rings.* It made me feel less afraid, steadier on my feet. I'd bring it home and put it by the back door."

"Like a talisman?" I asked.

"Yes. When I held them, I felt stronger, protected."

In an effort to rediscover the feeling of connectedness to nature on a more constant basis, Sam has started a hiking club with fellow med students. They take day trips, hike, and sometimes collect beautiful sticks, which they post photos of online, as part of a movement called Stick Nation. (Apparently, Sam is not the only one who appreciates the simple joy of finding and holding a stick that feels awe-inspiring when he clasps it in his hands.) In the photos Sam sends me, he and his friends stand on top of a rocky mountain promontory, holding their magnificent sticks aloft like Gandalf. Sam's eyes are alert, alight, as if he's reawakening some familiar, private joy within.

Paola and Will have also picked up a new hobby: salsa dancing. The goal is twofold: to enhance their ability to read each other's signals and communicate, and to stay active, but not with the kinds of sports and hobbies that Paola now finds too challenging. (No more spelunking for her!) As a child, Paola loved to dance; she took dance lessons until she went to college. "I stopped because everything became so performance-driven. I loved dancing, but not the competition. I'd have to fight off waves of dread before every performance." Salsa dancing with Will is different. It's intuitive. It's joyful. "It's changing our dynamic. We have to stay attuned to each other in every step. It's teaching us how to be gentle and encourage each other when one of us messes up, which we both do a lot. He's learning to lean into the teamwork required instead of throwing blame or mocking me. We're having real moments of joy together."

When Paola tells me this, I think of all we know about how our deepest emotional wounding happens in relationships. Sometimes our most profound healing occurs when it, too, happens in relationships.

Another acquaintance of mine, James, an engineer, has cleared out his garage and turned it into a carpentry workshop. He and his wife had recently become estranged from their son, and James found himself spending far too much of his time in mental rehearsals of his deep anguish about his son, who won't speak to them. He knew he needed to harness his energy in a more productive, life-affirming way. He decided to put it into designing and building bright, colorful furniture—bunk beds, chairs, tables—for children in homeless shelters. Creating these "tangible things in the world with my hands" has brought him "not just relief from dwelling in stories of what I could have done differently as a dad, it's made me feel I'm part of something larger, that there is still meaning to be found in my life."

From a neurobiological perspective, when we are engaged in hobbies for the sheer joy they offer, our creative brain circuitry becomes so active it prevents the circuitry that plunges the default mode network into rumination from happening. It's kind of like an old house where you can't use all the electrical circuits at once. (If you've ever lived in a house where you can't run the clothes dryer and the hair dryer at the same time without blowing a fuse, you know what I mean.) By engaging your creativity and imagination circuitry, you circumvent the circuitry that plunges you into rumination. All three areas of the default mode network are active, but they're no longer surging into overdrive. Instead, they're interfacing with the whole brain, allowing full, expansive—even transformative—creative ideation and awareness.

Minimize Unhealthy Distraction

Most of us are feeling overwhelmed by what's happening in our world, and it's hard to avoid getting sucked into scrolling and reading articles about what a dark time this is. But even if you want to remain an informed citizen, it's possible—more than possible, desirable—to do that and still choose to spend less time on your devices. If you want to move out of unhealthy rumination and into the upside of rumination, you are absolutely going to have to disconnect, at least every once in a while, from your phone, tablet, computer, social media apps, and any other entry into the digital world's rabbit hole. As philosopher and neuroscientist Sam Harris recently said, "There is a multi-front war being fought for our attention and most of us are losing it thanks to our devices."

Without needing to reference the thousands (tens of thousands?) of studies that tell us this, I think we all know that our weddedness to our phones is making it impossible for us to be fully present to ourselves or to the people we care most about. Photographer Eric Pickersgill brought this home in his project *Removed.* He photographed people staring at their phones—couples in bed together, kids sitting on sofas, people strolling in nature and walking down the street. He then removed the phones from the photographs so that all you see is people staring blankly with flat, zoned-out expressions into their empty palms, oblivious of themselves, each other, and the world.

Like so many of us, med student Sam wants to detach himself from technology. "I want to focus on what I want to focus on, and sometimes, I'll admit it, I can't fully do that when my phone is even in the room."

To help Sam put his phone far, far away and choose healthier pursuits, I share with him a 2025 study in which researchers at the University of Texas at Austin had 467 people put their phones away for two weeks. (Yes, I can see your eyebrows shooting up with incredulity at this suggestion, just as Sam's did.) Ninety-one percent of participants reported experiencing far better moods, taking more pleasure in life, spending more time in nature, engaging more in hobbies, feeling more socially connected, and being better able to focus and pay attention. In fact, the effects on mood were so profound, they were comparable to those seen with antidepressants. "I want that—if I can get myself to do it," Sam tells me. You can no doubt relate.

Maximize Healthy Distraction

Perhaps you remember the famous marshmallow study conducted at Stanford University in the 1970s. Researchers brought children between the ages of three and five into a room and presented them with a marshmallow. Then they gave each child a choice: They could eat their marshmallow right away, or, if they waited for fifteen minutes without eating it, they'd receive a second marshmallow as a reward. Kids wiggled and squirmed as they stared down the marshmallow, trying not to give in—but most did. Still, a few managed to wait the full time without taking even a nibble. Those kids who waited later, as teens, had higher SAT scores and showed more signs of achievement. They were also in better physical and mental health. The study led researchers to believe that the ability to delay gratification in childhood was a strong predictor of future life success.

But over time, researchers have fine-tuned this discussion, arguing that the kids who didn't eat the marshmallow weren't necessarily better at self-control, they were better at *distracting themselves* in fruitful ways. Instead of staring at the marshmallow when researchers left the room, they sang, talked to themselves, tapped their feet, made funny faces, or otherwise entertained themselves. By finding constructive ways to distract themselves, they avoided ruminating about or fixating on the marshmallow in front of them—which would have led to grabbing and gulping it down—and won their extra marshmallow reward.

Other research backs up the idea that healthy distraction helps us disengage from ruminative states. In one study, researchers purposely encouraged 102 young people to ruminate about something that distressed them until they were in a "negative mood." They then introduced different brief interventions for "stopping the ruminative process": distraction, problem-solving, and mindfulness strategies. Problem-solving—continuing to focus on what they were feeling, why they felt that way, and what they could do to avoid any negative consequences of the event they were ruminating on—was least likely to help them. Mindfulness skills helped. But here's what surprised me when I read this study: Introducing very brief periods of distraction in which their subjects thought about various simple and random things that the researchers suggested—like the shiny surface of a trumpet, or what the layout of the local shopping center looked like—was what most quickly alleviated ruminating thoughts. (This reminds me of a simple hack to help people fall asleep. You can distract yourself from fretful nighttime thoughts by taking an imaginary "house tour." Think of a house you know well, other than your own, and slowly walk up to the door. As you enter, notice the floors, the pictures on the walls, the furniture. Hopefully, to borrow from the work of Robert Louis Stevenson, you'll be in "the land of Nod" in no time.)

To use healthy distraction to your benefit, think of any absorbing activity you enjoy. The brain loves a goal to chase. Without a little direction from you, it will chase down the wrong paths in a misguided attempt to bring you relief. So give it something to chase that will feel good when you do it. A walk in nature, calling a friend you miss and haven't talked to in a long time, reading a book that you can't put down, putting on music and singing along, giving yourself a facial, going through old photos. It can be especially helpful to engage your hands (which helps your brain to refocus): Try a new bread recipe, create a flower arrangement, or clean out that cluttered kitchen junk drawer where you stuff your oddball doodads. Or you can re-practice any of the strategies you've learned in this book thus far—all of which qualify as, yes, very nourishing distraction.

A few weeks ago, I was at the beach off-season by myself. I was renting a place so I could have undisturbed time to, well, work on this book. As I walked alone on the beach, where I'd spent so many summer days with my children when they were young, I got caught up in past memories of the years when I was too sick to be the mother I wanted to be to my children and soothe their sense of terror over my long absences. My mind became momentarily trapped in its old shadowy corners—those whispered narratives of self-blame and regret.

But some part of me, having done the work to curb and repurpose my mind drama into something more open and transformative, was also speaking to me, wishing something better for me than self-flagellation. Suddenly, I began to sing as I walked along the beach. With no one else in sight, I sang as loudly as I could. I am not a good singer. I mean this. I cannot carry a tune. But still, I sang. I sang and sang and sang. Slowly, memories came back to me from before my father had died. How he and I had both loved to experiment and play with language and words, and how when he got home from his newspaper office, he'd encourage me to sing the songs I'd "written" that day. As five- and six-year-olds will, I'd sing out my little rhymes, my daffy songs, weaving in my stories from my day, totally unself-conscious because I could count on my father's delight in me.

And so I sang to the sea and to my long-ago self. Now, when I am by the sea, my new act of self-love is to find an isolated part of the beach where I can sing to the sea, and no one else can hear it—only the sea and me.

Drift with Your Thoughts When You First Wake Up

Another way to access the upside of rumination is to linger for a few precious moments (or longer if you can take the time) in that delicious liminal, transitional state between sleep and wakefulness. Paul Seli, PhD, assistant professor of psychology and neuroscience at the Duke Institute for Brain Sciences, is both neuroscientist and artist. He's shown that when we let our minds drift in this liminal half-asleep state, we experience a unique opportunity to discover new insights and answers to problems. The scientific term for this state is *hypnagogia.* In these dreamlike moments, we're "able to link things together that we normally wouldn't connect," Seli explains. For him, he says, "it's like there's an artist in my brain that I get to know through hypnagogia." To help capture these semi-lucid moments and any inspired ideas they give rise to, keep paper and pencil by your bed, and as you wake, jot everything down that comes to you. You may find there is a more creative person in your brain that you can get to know through these moments of hypnagogia.

In her novel *Creation Lake,* writer Rachel Kushner writes about such liminal moments. She calls these "states, hypnagogic or waking," our "invisible real." Here, "imagination and sleep and dreaming" become "the interwoven tresses of a single glossy braid." We become open to that "grand sense, of the heaven right here on earth; a garden of delights you should not wait for, pray for, but live in, occupy, and enjoy."

One strategy I use—created by LinkedIn founder Reid Hoffman—to help me benefit from this hypnagogic state is to give my mind an overnight task. If I'm struggling with a problem, before I go to sleep, I set the conundrum before my brain. It might be a problem I've encountered in my writing. It might be how to have that delicate conversation with someone I love. It might be a difficult decision I'm barreling toward that presents me with equally gnarly choices (this happens often when managing chronic health issues). Rather than try to resolve it (and stay awake ruminating), I turn the problem over to my subconscious by writing down the specific problem, idea, or challenge I want to solve (or resolve). Then I ask my mind to work on it while I sleep. It's extraordinary how useful this simple strategy often proves to be. When I wake up, I jot down whatever ideas or potential solutions have come to me, while my mind is still fresh and undistracted.

Even if no clear answer emerges, the lingering sense of being on the right path to an answer serves to wrap me in that hypnagogic state a little longer, so I can cocoon and simmer in an expanded sense of possibility. This often leads to a new sense of clarity, a new knowing about what feels most right. Either way, this feels like a win; a far more delicious way to begin the day than scrolling on my phone to see the latest grim headlines.

If you find it hard to access a hypnagogic state, start by writing down anything you can remember from your dreams. This simple act, repeated every morning, will allow your subconscious mind to break through to your conscious mind. As with all things related to neural plasticity, the more you do it, the more doable it becomes.

Make Time for Mind-Meandering

Simple daydreaming—letting your mind stretch and wander—also builds the capacity for more creative rumination. Here, it can help your brain rise to the occasion if you set aside a specific time of day to mind-meander. Bring paper and pencil. And if inspired, write down some of what passes through your daydreaming mind. Later, see if anything stands out to you as a thread you'd like to follow to see where it leads in your next mind-meandering session.

Or you might set aside time each day to give yourself mini creative challenges. Write in iambic pentameter. Craft a haiku in three minutes. Draw with your nondominant hand. Work on a crossword puzzle or do Wordle. Learn to knit. As you do small, stimulating creative practices, notice what time of day tends to foster your peak creativity and mental clarity. When do you get your best ideas? Set this time of day aside, every day, and cherish those moments. Your brain does.

Whatever road you choose into mind-wandering, carry your sketchbook or idea journal with you throughout the day. Once you start the wheels turning, more moments of insight will arrive. You want to be prepared to capture them.

Wander in Nature

You've heard this a thousand times before, so consider this your reminder. You need to walk, hike, skip, run, and wander more in nature. Neuroscientists have found that when we're immersed in nature, the default mode network is quicker to spark wonder and imagination.

The poet David Whyte captures this nature-inspired mindset beautifully in his poem "Twice Blessed." As he stood knee-deep in a flooded field, he writes, "I allowed myself to be astonished by the great everywhere calling to me." Whyte speaks to that universal experience in which nature becomes our portal to a vaster, more reflective state of being. Perhaps you, too, know that feeling, when the world—the music of birds, the gladness of trees, the sky, the clouds, the stars, the cosmos—seems to split you open, atom by atom, so that you dissolve into it and become one with it.

Combining walking with being in nature is a double win. In one study—no surprise—individuals who walked for five to eight minutes in nature showed significantly enhanced levels of creative thinking; their ability to generate new ideas increased by 60 percent. Steve Jobs often used walking as a strategic way to foster clear thinking. So did Aristotle. To use Nietzsche's words, "All truly great thoughts are conceived while walking." All of these creative thinkers were onto something. Walking in and of itself helps the brain to flip from rumination to ideation, in part because we're engaging in what's known as *bilateral stimulation*, which helps the brain switch from self-focused thinking to open-minded awareness.

The point here is that once you have cleared your mind of the fog and mist of your ruminations, you're so much closer to hearing your true inner voice. Or, better yet, to quote Mary Oliver, you can at last discover how you want to live "your one wild and precious life."

One reason that walking in nature decreases rumination is that nature fills us with such instant awe—that feeling we experience when we are in the presence of something far vaster than ourselves—that at least for those moments, we transcend whatever has been consuming us. Studies show this feeling of awe is crucial to our well-being, in the same way that love and joy are. Experiencing it also triggers the release of oxytocin, that feel-good hormone that promotes trust and a feeling of connection to others. In one study, researcher Dacher Keltner, a psychologist at UC Berkeley, found that when we experience awe, we activate our vagus nerve, which helps to relax us and to deepen our breathing. Awe stills that critical voice in our heads by "deactivating the default mode network," he showed. Awe removes us from our self-preoccupation and gets us out of our own heads so we "realize our place in the larger context, our communities."

Another study showed that college students who experienced higher levels of awe felt a greater sense of empathy and connection to others and were more likely to volunteer to help others. I think anything that makes us more likely to reach out to, connect with, and look out for one another is something we need a lot more of right now.

Many of us, Keltner found, have two or three such awe experiences a week—and if we make a point of immersing ourselves in them as they unfold, we will continue to feel their reverberations in the days that follow. One way to find more awe in your life and become more conscious of it is to keep an awe journal and write down those special moments. Later, look back and see if you notice patterns. You could learn something about yourself and about what you might want to spend more time on: You love reading aloud to small children and witnessing their giggles and joy, so perhaps you want to volunteer to read to children at the local library or hospital; or your most profound moments of awe occur when hiking, so you join a hiking club; or you are filled with a sense of transcendence when witnessing acts of kindness by others, which could inspire you to make a commitment to offer some kind of compassionate gesture every day—something as modest as bringing in the mail for the elderly neighbor you saw struggling down the driveway to the mailbox, sending an email birthday greeting to someone you've been out of touch with for a long time, or making the time to give a tourist directions even when you're in a rush to get somewhere.

Whatever opens you to awe, do more of it. Recently, I was driving down a country road, on my way home from an appointment with yet another doctor, about yet another treatment she thought I should start, and I was thought-spiraling without even being aware that I was doing it. However, as I took a familiar winding turn in the road, the setting sun seemed to suddenly skip and drop in its dramatic descent into nothingness, sending one final yellow flare up. The car filled with an explosion of soft orange light that seemed to radiate straight into my bones. It brought my thought spirals to a sudden halt. Even though it had to have been an optical illusion, it was so unusual a sight that I gasped. I had driven that road for fifteen years and had never seen the sun disappear like that, as if it offered a portal opening to another world—a world in which all was healed. I felt, in that moment, as if nature were speaking directly to me, sending me a message about the extraordinary beauty that could be mine every day if only I would look for it.

The next day, I left my attic office and went outside at that same time of day, and there it was again, a sun that seemed to drop its light—and its lightness—into my whole being. It was almost spring, and each following day, when I went out to watch the moment of sunset, it arrived a minute or two later. Making a daily habit of going out to meet that end-of-day sun freed me from my thoughts and filled me with gratitude for the riches that surround us.

However you access your Inner Muse, I hope you do so with a sense of delight for the opportunity to create a time, a portal, a space that is just for you. Whenever my mind returns to its perseverations about all the usual subjects, I try to think of what artist René Magritte once wrote about creating enchantment: "Life is wasted when we make it more terrifying, precisely because it is so easy to do so. . . . Creating enchantment is an effective means of counteracting this depressing, banal habit." Let your Inner Muse usher you toward that enchantment, whenever and wherever you can.

CONCLUSION

WHEN I RETURN to Mark Trullinger to see what's happening in my brain, here is what I learn. After hooking me up to the wizardry of his machinery, Trullinger asks me to tell him about whatever feels most pressing in my life right now. It takes me a few minutes to find something that feels difficult. There is no interior litany of what's wrong and why running through my mind. This in and of itself feels entirely new. *Is this,* I ask myself, *because things in my life are going more swimmingly?* No, that's not it. Life was still doing what life does, presenting its ever-changing string of problems.

Trullinger asks me instead about a few things that I have, in the past, found challenging to talk about: tricky relationships in my extended family and of course my health. As he questions me and I recount a few incidents and bits of news that, in different form, could make up any human life, I realize I feel . . . calm. Perhaps even . . . relaxed, contemplative.

"This is good," Trullinger says, watching the computer screen, which I cannot see. "You're not slipping into rumination, even when your thoughts veer into territory that's been challenging for you in the past. But the real question is: What are you experiencing? How do you *feel?*"

As I take stock of my mental, ruminating life, it's clear, I tell Trullinger, that, on some primal level, my mind is less agitated, less likely to spit forth narratives that hook me into fear, resentment, or stories of my own unworthiness. At the same time, my proximity to creativity and imagination, my open-mindedness and sense of connectedness to myself and others, feels more concrete and expansive.

"Has your attention, your memory, improved?"

"I think it has," I tell him. I described how I felt more able to hold the multiple dancing threads of an idea in my mind and play with them, then set them down and pick them up again hours or days later, even after having been interrupted by big life events.

Still, I am curious to know, "How's the default mode network looking?"

"Quite different from when you had your first brain assessment." Trullinger tells me that my default mode network is no longer hyperactivated; it's connecting to my whole brain in a more integrated way. "This tells me you're able to meet whatever difficulties you're facing with greater emotional freedom." Trullinger pauses. "Better yet, you're holding this state, you don't show signs of slipping out of it. When you start to veer toward rumination, you're able to pull yourself back again."

"Are there still other anomalies in my brain?"

"Yes. But that's a good thing. You don't want a perfectly 'normal brain.' A brain that meets the norm in every kind of way—that's usually a brain that doesn't have quite as much potential. The thing that makes each of us so interesting is our beautiful abnormalities. It's just a matter of harnessing those in the right way. Those beautiful abnormalities are what make us capable of the most extraordinary things."

I hope, having tried the ideas we've explored together, you are feeling more *you.* I hope you have come to see that all you have experienced, carried, persevered through, has paved the way to a new understanding of, and liberation from, all that no longer serves you. The simple truth—writ inside our ruminations—is that we grow not by avoiding what gives rise to our pain but by engaging with it with curiosity and compassion. The places in us that we once held as shameful, the moments in which we were most egregiously misunderstood, made afraid, or deeply wounded, become the pattern in the fabric of our stories, and in these stories, we find—if we look for them—sacred gifts. Each moment of seeing and knowing ourselves, and finally waking up on our own side, is a hard-won puzzle piece representing a small but important victory. The powerful invitation here is to embrace the complexity of your story and bring forth the precious pieces of your psyche that are waiting to be seen, brought to light, understood—and revered.

When we do this, when we finally let go of anything we've been holding on to, or white knuckling, when we honor and attend to both the depth of our pain and our longing for peace, our minds register and respond to this. Our brains begin to hum together in a synchronized way. Everything feels easier. Hard things aren't quite so hard.

As I leave you, I hope you stand at the doorway of something wonderful—that you feel more seen, including by yourself, more loving, especially toward yourself, more attuned to inspiration and insight, and a bit braver as you continue your journey. From this gentle, strong space, I hope you take more delight in yourself—that core, elemental you—and in the world.

Wherever you are, however it's going, today, tomorrow, I want you to know there is magic in you, and I hope you see it now, too.

APPENDIX

Are You Ruminating Too Much?

TRY AS YOU MIGHT, you can't draw on the power of your whole, glorious brain when your default mode network has locked down into a state of rumination. If you're wondering whether you are inclined to get caught up in unhealthy rumination more than is good for you, this simple ten-minute questionnaire will shed some light on that.

In consultation with experts, including Ruth Lanius, MD, PhD, professor of psychiatry at the Western University of Canada and one of the leading neuroscientists who studies how the default mode network is shaped by life experiences, and inspired by questionnaires used to assess our proclivity to ruminate, I developed this quiz to serve as a tool for simple self-inquiry. But unlike other such questionnaires, it is not meant to offer you a score or a "diagnosis." There's no "if you answered yes to more than ten of these questions, then . . ." conclusion to be drawn here about your mental health, or lack thereof. What this quiz can do is help you to think about what rumination actually looks like in daily life and how much of it you do. The goal here is to help you discern if unwanted patterns of rumination and overthinking are fueling distress in your life, and if so, whether this is something you'd like to work on.

Read the following statements and decide which of them apply to you. As you do so, think about some of the concerns you've had about difficult experiences in the past, or even as recently as yesterday, and whether these are playing a role in your ruminations.

Answer a simple "Agree, that's me" (or a simple check mark will do) or "Disagree, that's not me" (or a simple *x* will do) to each of the following statements:

1. The same thoughts keep going through my mind again and again.

2. I find myself reliving certain memories or events from the past, unable to let go of them.

3. I can't stop mentally rehashing conversations that happened days, weeks, or years ago, thinking about what I could have said or should have said.

4. I often feel as though I don't have control over the thoughts that come into my mind.

5. I often find myself dwelling on past events or worrying about what the future holds.

6. Long after I've had an argument with someone, my thoughts keep going back to it.

7. I often lie awake at night, replaying scenes that upset me during the day.

8. I find myself constantly questioning decisions I made in the past.

9. My thoughts get in the way of paying attention to the things I need to focus on right now.

10. I spend too much time wondering and worrying about what others think of me.

11. I tend to dwell on things people said or did to me for a long time afterward.

12. When making choices, I tend to overanalyze and get stuck in indecision.

13. I often feel mentally exhausted or unable to relax.

14. Long stretches of time pass before I realize I've been caught up in my thoughts.

15. Sometimes it is hard for me to shut off negative thoughts about myself.

16. I often try to imagine what would have happened if events had gone differently in the past.

17. I keep second-guessing my decisions and wondering if they were mistakes.

18. I spend a great deal of time thinking back over my most embarrassing or disappointing moments.

19. My mind often imagines the worst that could happen.

20. I feel a strong need to know what the future holds and have difficulty with uncertainty.

Remember: You are not scoring or judging yourself here. Evaluating the relevance of these statements is merely a tool for honest self-inquiry, to help you see if rumination is a common habit for you. That said, if you agreed with most of these statements, you are likely experiencing rumination more than is good for you—which you probably already knew, even if you hadn't put a name to it or identified it as problematic. If you agreed with many of them, you are probably overthinking more than you want to. If you disagreed with most, lucky you! You're probably among that rare group of people who are not problem ruminators.

For those who agreed with most or many of these statements, however, know we're in this together. Most of us are ruminating far more than we want to or than is good for us. Happily, the latest annals of neuroscience offer extraordinary amounts of information about how to transform rumination from a reflex into a resource for reflection, insight, and growth—which is the subject of this book, which you now hold in your hands.

ACKNOWLEDGMENTS

I COULDN'T HAVE written this book without the help of three extraordinary women. My agent, Elizabeth Kaplan, has stalwartly stood by my side through every iteration of every big book idea I've ever had. My beloved editor, Marnie Cochran, with whom I've worked for most of my career, never fails to make the writing process feel like joyful teamwork. And for this book, I'm particularly indebted to Ruth Lanius, MD, PhD, professor of psychiatry, the Harris-Woodman Chair in Mind-Body Medicine, and director of the Clinical Research Program for PTSD at the Western University of Canada, who graciously served as my guide through much of the journey recounted in these pages, proving to be a treasure house of information, both practical and theoretical.

I'm also indebted to the many experts who spent time with me in person and on Zoom, especially Mark Trullinger and Jessica Christie-Sands. A heartfelt thanks, too, to John Cammack and Henry Harbin, of BrainFutures, for their advice on new and promising offerings in the world of neurotechnology.

To my early draft readers, Shannon Brownlee and Peggy Orenstein, thank you for your keen, helpful insights (not to mention your friendship). And I especially want to thank Beth Rashbaum, who read and worked on my earliest draft and helped me discern what really needed to be in these pages, versus what parts could go. She made this a better book.

But the most important thanks go to the many individuals who trusted me with their stories. You may be disguised, but you know who you are. I thank you for allowing me to share your experiences. I might have been the writer, but you quickly became my teachers.

For me, the act of creating and writing only feels right, and goes swimmingly, when I'm surrounded by my family and friends, because nothing else really matters. To my husband, Zen, and my children, Christian and Claire, you put the magic in this journey we are all on together.

NOTES

Preface

xiv **Nearly twenty thousand people:** The Sesame Street social media account @Elmo posted this on X on January 29, 2024.

xiv **In a quickly released statement:** Callie Holterman, "Elmo Asked an Innocuous Question," *New York Times*, January 30, 2024.

Chapter 1: The Power and Peril of Rumination

7 **Compared to prior to the pandemic:** M. Xiao et al., "Stronger Functional Network Connectivity and Social Support Buffer Against Negative Affect During the COVID-19 Outbreak and After the Pandemic Peak," *Neurobiology of Stress* 15 (November 2021): 100418. In this study, researchers found that our feelings of "negative affect" increased during the pandemic and did not decrease after the pandemic, and these changes in negative emotional response and regulation processes were associated with alterations of three brain regions, including the default mode network. N. Pan et al., "Pre-COVID Brain Functional Connectome Features Prospectively Predict Emergence of Distress Symptoms After Onset of the COVID-19 Pandemic," *Psychological Medicine* 53, no. 11 (2023): 5155–66; X. Liu et al., "Psychological Resilience Mediates the Protective Role of Default-Mode Network Functional Connectivity Against COVID-19 Vicarious Traumatization," *Translational Psychiatry* 13, no. 1 (2023): 231;

S. Dubey et al., "The Cognitive Basis of Psychosocial Impact in COVID-19 Pandemic. Does It Encircle the Default Mode Network of the Brain? A Pragmatic Proposal," *Medical Research Archives* 10, no. 3 (2022): 10.18103.

7 **And yup, most of us appear to be:** J. W. Fredrick et al., "Rumination as a Mechanism of the Longitudinal Association Between COVID-19-Related Stress and Internalizing Symptoms in Adolescents," *Child Psychiatry and Human Development* 55, no. 2 (2024): 531–40; D. B. O'Connor et al., "Effects of COVID-19-Related Worry and Rumination on Mental Health and Loneliness During the Pandemic: Longitudinal Analyses of Adults in the UK-COVID-19 Mental Health & Wellbeing Study," *Journal of Mental Health* 32, no. 6 (2023): 1122–33.

7 **Everything we could possibly stew:** This quote is based on my emails with psychologist Sally Winston, PsyD, on January 23, 2025.

8 **And most of this rumination time:** Steve Bradt, "Wandering Mind Not a Happy Mind," *Harvard Gazette*, November 11, 2010.

8 **Today, 20 percent of U.S. adults:** "Anxiety and Depression: Household Pulse Survey," Centers for Disease Control and Prevention, National Center for Health Statistics, 2024; "Estimates of Mental Health Symptomatology, by Month of Interview: United States," Centers for Disease Control and Prevention, National Center for Health Statistics, 2019. For statistics showing that in 2024 between 20.7 and 22.2 percent of adults reported symptoms of depression or anxiety: https://www.cdc.gov/nchs/covid19/pulse/mental-health.htm (see drop-down menu for "Symptoms of Anxiety Disorder or Depressive Disorder"). To compare 2024 statistics to 2019 statistics, which showed that 9.5 to 11.7 percent of adults reported symptoms of anxiety or depression: https://www.cdc.gov/nchs/data/nhis/mental-health-monthly-508.pdf.

8 **Only one in three U.S. adults:** Megan Brenan, "Americans' Reported Mental Health at New Low; More Seek Help," Gallup, December 21, 2022, https://news.gallup.com/poll/467303/americans-reported-mental-health-new-low-seek-help.aspx.

8 **And in 2024, the Gallup World Poll:** Allison Aubrey, "U.S. Drops in New Global Happiness Ranking. One Age Group Bucks the Trend," NPR, March 20, 2024, https://www.npr.org/sections/health-shots/2024/03/20/1239537074/u-s-drops-in-new-global-happiness-ranking-one-age-group-bucks-the-trend.

8 **Perhaps one reason why answering:** J. M. Newby et al., "Understanding the Experience of Rumination and Worry: A Descriptive Qualitative Survey Study," *British Journal of Clinical Psychology* 61, no. 4 (2022): 929–46.

9 **It's hard to solve a problem:** Y. Xie et al., "Perfectionism, Worry, Rumination, and Distress: A Meta-analysis of the Evidence for the Per-

fectionism Cognition Theory," *Personality and Individual Differences* 139 (March 2019): 301–12.

9 **According to *Merriam-Webster*:** *Merriam-Webster Dictionary*, "ruminate," https://www.merriam-webster.com/dictionary/ruminate.

10 **A well-functioning mind:** Maria Popova quotes Alain de Botton in her blog, "Alain de Botton on the Qualities of a Healthy Mind," *The Marginalian*, October 25, 2023, https://www.themarginalian.org/2023/10/25/alain-de-botton-healthy-mind/.

Chapter 2: Why We Ruminate—and the Price We Pay

13 **She studied for her PhD:** "In Memoriam: Susan Nolen-Hoeksema," *Yale News*, January 7, 2013, https://news.yale.edu/2013/01/07/memoriam-susan-nolen-hoeksema; S. Lyubomirsky et al., "Thinking About Rumination: The Scholarly Contributions and Intellectual Legacy of Susan Nolen-Hoeksema," *Annual Review of Clinical Psychology* 11 (January 2015): 1–22.

13 **Confronted by a bad situation:** Martin Seligman, *Learned Optimism* (Alfred A. Knopf, 1991). Also see Maria Popova, "Learned Optimism: Martin Seligman on Happiness, Depression, and the Meaningful Life," *The Marginalian*, June 28, 2012, https://www.themarginalian.org/2012/06/28/learned-optimism-martin-seligman/.

13 **Or, as Seligman puts it:** Seligman, *Learned Optimism.*

13 **She was interested in:** Lyubomirsky et al., "Thinking About Rumination." Nolen-Hoeksema's graduate research at first focused on understanding predictors of depression among children and adolescents. She examined learned helplessness, pessimism, and adverse life experiences in the development of depression. This led her to her research examining rumination as a risk factor in depression—something she found to be truer for girls than for boys.

14 **She described rumination as:** "Most Women Think Too Much, Overthinkers Often Drink Too Much," University of Michigan News, February 4, 2003, https://news.umich.edu/most-women-think-too-much-overthinkers-often-drink-too-much/. This press release defines Susan Nolen-Hoeksema's concept of rumination as "endless torrents of negative thoughts and emotions." Also see Susan Nolen-Hoeksema, *Women Who Think Too Much* (Henry Holt, 2003).

14 **Your brain becomes so caught up:** Lyubomirsky et al., "Thinking About Rumination."

14 **Often, Nolen-Hoeksema found:** "Most Women Think Too Much," *University of Michigan News;* Nolen-Hoeksema, *Women Who Think Too Much.*

15 **In William Shakespeare's comedy:** William Shakespeare, *As You Like It*, in *William Shakespeare Complete Works*, ed. Jonathan Bate and Eric Rasmussen (Modern Library, 2022), 501.

15 **Russian novelist Fyodor Dostoevsky:** Fyodor Dostoevsky, *Notes from Underground*, trans. Jessie Coulson (Penguin, 1972), 17.

15 **The constant analysis of our:** Fyodor Dostoevsky, *Notes from Underground*, trans. Richard Pevear and Larissa Volokhonsky (Vintage, 1993), 43.

15 **Left unchecked, a routinely ruminating mind:** Lyubomirsky et al., "Thinking About Rumination."

15 **Following up on Nolen-Hoeksema's research:** X. Xu, H. Yuan, and X. Lei, "Activation and Connectivity within the Default Mode Network Contribute Independently to Future-Oriented Thought," *Scientific Reports* 12, no. 6 (2016): 21001; X. Chen et al., "Rumination and the Default Mode Network: Meta-analysis of Brain Imaging Studies and Implications for Depression," *NeuroImage* 206 (February 2020): 116287.

15 **In a 2023 study using fMRI:** J. Kim et al., "A Dorsomedial Prefrontal Cortex–Based Dynamic Functional Connectivity Model of Rumination," *Nature Communications* 14, no. 1 (2023): 3540.

16 **Other studies have shown that:** D. Pan et al., "Emotional Working Memory Training Reduces Rumination and Alters the EEG Microstate in Anxious Individuals," *NeuroImage: Clinical* 28 (November 2020): 102488; T. Onraedt and E. H. W. Koster, "Training Working Memory to Reduce Rumination," *PLOS One* 9, no. 3 (2014): e90632.

16 **And researchers who study Alzheimer's:** G. Koch et al., "Precuneus Magnetic Stimulation for Alzheimer's Disease: A Randomized, Sham-Controlled Trial," *Brain* 145, no. 11 (2022): 3776–86.

16 **The degree of our tendency to ruminate:** R. A. Sansone and L. A. Sansone, "Rumination: Relationships with Physical Health," *Innovations in Clinical Neuroscience* 9, no. 2 (2012): 29–34.

17 **Many, if not most, of us:** "More Than a Quarter of U.S. Adults Say They're So Stressed They Can't Function," American Psychological Association, October 19, 2022, https://www.apa.org/news/press/releases/2022/10/multiple-stressors-no-function.

17 **Among youth ages eighteen to thirty-four:** Anna Medaris, "Gen Z Adults and Younger Millennials Are 'Completely Overwhelmed' by Stress," American Psychological Association, November 1, 2023, https://www.apa.org/topics/stress/generation-z-millennials-young-adults-worries.

17 **In a study released in 2025:** "Sapien Releases the Mental State of the World Report for 2024," Sapien Labs, February 28, 2025, https://

sapienlabs.org/whats_new/sapien-releases-the-mental-state-of-the-world-report-for-2024/.

17 **Among high school students:** "2023 Youth Risk Behavior Survey Results," Centers for Disease Control and Prevention, Youth Risk Behavior Surveillance System, September 29, 2024, https://www.cdc.gov/yrbs/results/2023-yrbs-results.html; "U.S. Teen Girls Experiencing Increased Sadness and Violence," CDC Newsroom, February 13, 2023, https://www.cdc.gov/media/releases/2023/p0213-yrbs.html.

17 **It's little wonder that:** Jonathan Haidt, "Why the Mental Health of Liberal Girls Sank First and Fastest," *Free Press*, March 13, 2023.

18 **Professor Susan David, PhD:** Susan David, "The Gift and Power of Emotional Courage," TED video, 17:48, November 2017, https://www.ted.com/talks/susan_david_the_gift_and_power_of_emotional_courage?language=en.

Chapter 3: A Hidden Desire Behind Our Mind Drama

23 **At the Institute for Early Life Adversity:** E. T. C. Lippard and C. B. Nemeroff, "The Devastating Clinical Consequences of Child Abuse and Neglect: Increased Disease Vulnerability and Poor Treatment Response in Mood Disorders," *American Journal of Psychiatry* 177, no. 1 (2020): 20–36; Stephen M. Strakowski, "The 'Single Biggest Contributor' to Medical and Mental Illness," *Medscape*, January 24, 2020, https://www.medscape.com/viewarticle/923389.

24 **In its 2024 report:** E. A. Swedo et al., "Adverse Childhood Experiences and Health Conditions and Risk Behaviors Among High School Students—Youth Risk Behavior Survey, United States, 2023," *Morbidity and Mortality Weekly Report (MMWR)* 73, no. 4 (2024): 39–49.

24 **Researchers who study the adolescent brain:** T. C. Ho et al., "Emotion-Dependent Functional Connectivity of the Default Mode Network in Adolescent Depression," *Biological Psychiatry* 78, no. 9 (2015): 635–46.

25 **This echoes findings:** S. Lyubomirsky et al., "Effects of Ruminative and Distracting Responses to Depressed Mood on Retrieval of Autobiographical Memories," *Journal of Personality and Social Psychology* 75, no. 1 (1998): 166–77.

25 **These memories and montages:** J. M. Newby et al., "Understanding the Experience of Rumination and Worry: A Descriptive Qualitative Survey Study," *British Journal of Clinical Psychology* 61, no. 4 (2022): 929–46; B. E. Wisco and S. Nolen-Hoeksema, "Valence of Autobiographical Memories: The Role of Mood, Cognitive Reappraisal, and Suppression," *Behaviour Research and Therapy* 48, no. 4 (2010): 335–40.

26 **We are, to quote the poet Adrienne Rich:** Ed Pavlic, "Adrienne Rich's Solitudes," *Boston Review*, May 26, 2021.

26 **That entanglement showed up:** J. M. Newby et al., "Understanding the Experience."

26 **We often assume trauma:** Ed Tronick and Claudia M. Gold, *The Power of Discord: Why the Ups and Downs of Relationships Are the Secret to Building Intimacy, Resilience, and Trust* (Little, Brown, 2020).

29 **In one 2022 study, researchers:** T. Tian et al., "Default Mode Network Alterations Induced by Childhood Trauma Correlate with Emotional Function and SLCA4 Expression," *Frontiers in Psychiatry* 12 (January 2022): 760411.

30 **Adversity in childhood alters:** M. H. Teicher and J. A. Samson, "Annual Research Review: Enduring Neurobiological Effects of Childhood Abuse and Neglect," *Journal of Child Psychology and Psychiatry* 57, no. 3 (2016): 241–66.

32 **They found that even with minimal:** H. Hoffman et al., "Children with Maltreatment Exposure Exhibit Rumination-Like Spontaneous Thought Patterns: Association with Symptoms of Depression, Subcallosal Cingulate Cortex Thickness, and Cortisol Levels," *Journal of Childhood Psychology and Psychiatry, with Allied Disciplines* 65, no. 1 (2024): 31–41. In this study, researchers showed that children who experienced early life adversity showed changes in thickness in the subcallosal cingulate cortex (SCC) and cited a body of research showing that these changes in the SCC also influenced the SCC's functional connectivity to the default mode network and the frontoparietal network in ways that increase "depressive rumination."

32 **In a separate study of nearly six hundred:** B. Alligood et al., "Rumination as a Moderator of the Relation Between Childhood Adversity Exposure and College Students' Psychological Distress," *Journal of Trauma Studies in Education* 3, no. 2 (2024): 45–68. Also see J. Wang et al., "Childhood Trauma and Depressive Level Among Chinese College Students in Guangzhou: The Roles of Rumination and Perceived Stress," *Psychiatry Investigation* 21, no. 4 (2024): 352–60. And see C. Popielarz, "Neuroticism and Rumination as Mechanisms by Which Adverse Childhood Experiences Increase Vulnerability to Depression in College Students" (master's thesis, West Chester University, 2024), 328.

32 **Nolen-Hoeksema found similar evidence:** S. Nolen-Hoeksema et al., "Rumination as a Mechanism Linking Stressful Life Events to Symptoms of Depression and Anxiety: Longitudinal Evidence in Early Adolescents and Adults," *Journal of Abnormal Psychology* 122, no. 2 (2013): 339–52.

Chapter 4: Seeing Through Your Mind Drama

42 **According to psychologist Sally Winston:** Kate Kelly, "Don't Let Rumination Ruin Your Day," HealthCentral, June 5, 2023, https://www.healthcentral.com/condition/anxiety/rumination.

44 **You might borrow words of wisdom from Cher:** Jancee Dunn, "The Best Advice I've Ever Heard for How to Be Happy," *New York Times*, April 28, 2025.

46 **This is when all the parts of your brain:** For a deeper, more scientific understanding of how life adversity can impair neural connections and integration between key areas of the brain, including the default mode network, prefrontal cortex, orbitofrontal cortex, corpus callosum, hippocampus, and amygdala, and keep us from feeling whole, see M. H. Teicher and J. A. Samson, "Annual Research Review: Enduring Neurobiological Effects of Childhood Abuse and Neglect," *Journal of Child Psychology and Psychiatry* 57, no. 3 (2016): 241–66; and M. H. Teicher et al., "Recognizing the Importance of Childhood Maltreatment as a Critical Factor in Psychiatric Diagnoses, Treatment, Research, Prevention, and Education," *Molecular Psychiatry* 27 (November 2021): 1331–38.

46 **Though he says that for as:** This is drawn from Maria Popova's essay "How People Change: Psychoanalyst Allen Wheelis on the Essence of Freedom and the Two Elements of Self-Transcendence," *The Marginalian*, July 4, 2023, https://www.themarginalian.org/2023/07/04/allen-wheelis-how-people-change/.

Chapter 5: What Messages Are Your Ruminations Sending You?

54 **The poet Rumi once wrote:** Jalal al-Din Rumi, *The Essential Rumi*, trans. Coleman Barks (Castle Books, 1995), 80.

54 **For most of us, the answer is:** Oliver Burkeman, "Think You're Self-Aware? Think Again," *The Guardian*, May 26, 2017.

54 **"The effort of turning away one's thoughts":** Bertrand Russell, *The Conquest of Happiness* (W. W. Norton, 1996), 64.

56 **This idea of naming emotions:** J. B. Torre and M. D. Lieberman, "Putting Feelings into Words: Affect Labeling as Implicit Emotion Regulation," *Emotion Review* 10, no. 2 (2018): 116–24.

57 **When we "consciously appraise":** Ruth A. Lanius et al., *Sensory Pathways to Healing from Trauma: Harnessing the Brain's Capacity for Change* (Guilford Press, 2025), 10–11.

63 **Georgia O'Keeffe once wrote:** "Georgia O'Keeffe Quotes," Georgia O'Keeffe (website), https://www.georgiaokeeffe.org/quotes/.

63 **As Steve Jobs said:** Anthony D. Fredericks, "The Best Creativity Advice from Steve Jobs," *Psychology Today,* June 20, 2024.

63 **Physician and trauma expert:** Gabor Maté, MD, expresses this idea in his book *When the Body Says No: Understanding the Stress-Disease Connection* (J. Wiley & Sons, 2003).

63 **Or, to put it in Brené Brown's words:** Maryn Liles, "50 Brené Brown Quotes for Powerful Motivation," *Reader's Digest,* September 19, 2024.

Chapter 6: Your Understory

64 **In one 2017 study of students:** Joaquin Selva, "What Is Albert Ellis' ABC Model in CBT Theory?," *Positive Psychology,* March 8, 2018. Also see G. A. Saelid and H. M. Nordahl, "Rational Emotive Behaviour Therapy in High Schools to Educate in Mental Health and Empower Youth Health. A Randomized Controlled Study of a Brief Intervention," *Cognitive Behaviour Therapy* 46, no. 3 (2017): 196–210.

64 **Ripley says if you're unsure:** "Amanda Ripley: Stepping out of 'the Zombie Dance' We're In, and into 'Good Conflict' That Is, in Fact, Life-Giving," *On Being with Krista Tippett,* February 9, 2023; "Conflict Is Normal. Here's How to Keep It Healthy and Avoid Disaster / Amanda Ripley," *10% Happier with Dan Harris,* October 14, 2024.

70 **We know we have the tools:** Jonathan Haidt speaks to the importance of feeling one has a sense of agency and control over one's mental state, versus viewing oneself as fragile and powerless, in his essay "Why the Mental Health of Liberal Girls Sank First and Fastest," *Free Press,* March 13, 2023. In this essay, he talks about how important this is for young people in particular.

73 **Our heart rates slow as:** S. E. Taylor et al., "Biobehavioral Responses to Stress in Females: Tend-and-Befriend, Not Fight-or-Flight," *Psychological Review* 107, no. 3 (2000): 411–29.

73 **Replaying our injuries with friends:** J. S. Spendelow et al., "The Relationship Between Co-rumination and Internalizing Problems: A Systematic Review and Meta-analysis," *Clinical Psychology & Psychotherapy* 24, no. 2 (2017): 512–27.

77 **"A trap is only a trap":** China Mieville, *King Rat* (Macmillan, 2005), 254.

Chapter 7: Ballistic Interruption

81 **Luckily, there are new:** In addition to hearing this term used in the manufacturing and defense world to refer to a protective safety fea-

ture, I also heard the term *ballistic process interruption* used by Sarah Baldeo, in reference to "ballistic processes"—rapid, automatic, and unconscious neural or behavioral responses to stress or threat, in her 2023 TEDx Talk, "Neuroscience of Resilience: Ballistic Process Interruption," YouTube video, 18:37, posted by TEDx Talks, November 2, 2023, https://www.youtube.com/watch?v=XGe0cEGOjdE.

83 **Here are a few to try:** My interest in using self-commands to interrupt rumination began at a 2017 conference when I was giving a keynote at the Royal Society of Medicine, in London, hosted by the Stress Illness Recovery Practitioners' Association (SIRPA). One of the speakers was Georgie Oldfield, a physical therapist and founder of SIRPA. Oldfield spoke about methods for interrupting thoughts when you experience chronic pain. Neuroscientists have shown that *nociceptors*—nerve endings in skin, joints, and muscles—send signals to the brain that first trigger the sensation of pain. (The word *nociceptor* comes from the Latin word for "hurt.") If pain is chronic, over time, pain signals create neural pathways that create a feedback loop between body and mind. These pathways can become so established that nociceptors signal your brain you're in pain even when your body is healthy. This mind-body feedback loop that results in physical pain is exacerbated when we suppress or ignore our emotional pain. Physician John Sarno introduced this idea—that the more we sublimate our feelings, the more pain we have and the longer it sticks around—in the 1990s in his book *Healing Back Pain.* Other experts who use this methodology include Howard Schubiner, MD, author of *Unlearn Your Pain*, and physical therapist Cathleen King, DPT, founder of the mind-body program Primal Trust. Neuroscientists have since demonstrated that emotional and physical pain travel into our conscious awareness along the same neural pathways and that by treating our emotional wounds, we lessen physical pain. For this reason, pain specialists today often treat physical pain by asking you to address your emotional pain, too. One of the most successful ways to begin is by interrupting the negative thought loops, words, and feelings that fuel that brain-nociceptor feedback loop—a process called *neuromodulation.* For more on how emotional and chronic pain are intertwined, see N. Eisenberger, "The Pain of Social Disconnection: Examining the Shared Neural Underpinnings of Physical and Social Pain," *Nature Reviews Neuroscience* 13, no. 6 (2012): 421–34; C. N. Dewall et al., "Acetaminophen Reduces Social Pain: Behavioral and Neural Evidence," *Psychological Science* 21, no. 7 (2010): 931–37.

85 **Experimental psychologist Ethan Kross:** E. Kross et al., "Third-Person Self-Talk Facilitates Emotion Regulation Without Engaging Cognitive Control: Converging Evidence from ERP and fMRI," *Scientific Reports* 7, no. 1 (2017): 4519.

86 **Talking to yourself in the third person:** Ethan Kross, *Chatter* (Crown, 2021), 70.

86 **In a 2015 *New York Times* interview:** Brooks Barnes, "Jennifer Lawrence Has No Appetite for Playing Fame Games," *New York Times*, September 9, 2015.

86 **Studies looking at the language:** "Analysis of Social Media Language Using AI Models Predicts Depression Severity for White Americans, but Not Black Americans," National Institutes of Health, March 26, 2024, https://irp.nih.gov/news-and-events/in-the-news/analysis-of-social-media-language-using-ai-models-predicts-depression.

Chapter 8: Body-State Breakers

94 **The wife thinks:** Lorrie Moore, *Anagrams* (Vintage, 1986), 128.

96 **"Anybody who gets put down":** Instagram video, Gottman Institute (@gottmaninstitute), October 4, 2024.

96 **In his book *When the Body Says No:*** Gabor Maté, *When the Body Says No: Understanding the Stress-Disease Connection* (John Wiley & Sons, 2003), xi.

96 **Neuroscientists recently mapped:** B. S. McEwen and M. Picard, "Psychological Stress and Mitochondria: A Conceptual Framework," *Psychosomatic Medicine* 80, no. 2 (2018): 126–40.

97 **Your cells respond as if:** R. K. Naviaux, "Perspective: Cell Danger Response Biology—The New Science That Connects Environmental Health with Mitochondria and the Rising Tide of Chronic Illness," *Mitochondrion* 51 (March 2020): 40–45, https://doi.org/10.1016/j.mito.2019.12.005.

98 **This can be especially true:** X. Zhong et al., "Childhood Maltreatment Experience Influences Neural Response to Psychosocial Stress in Adults: An fMRI Study," *Frontiers in Psychology* 10 (January 2020): 2961.

101 **Your brain can't direct your muscles:** For more on this, see Thomas Hanna, *Somatics: Reawakening the Mind's Control of Movement, Flexibility, and Health* (Da Capo Press, 1988).

102 **According to Paul Conti:** Andrew Huberman, host, *Huberman Lab*, podcast, "Therapy, Treating Trauma & Other Life Challenges | Dr. Paul Conti," Scicomm Media, June 6, 2022.

103 **Individuals who practiced cyclic sighing:** Jenny Taitz, "The Positive Power of a Good Sigh," *Washington Post*, July 1–2, 2023; M. Y. Balban et al., "Brief Structured Respiration Practices Enhance Mood and Reduce Physiological Arousal," *Cell Reports: Medicine* 4, no. 1 (2023): 100895.

104 **It's designed to activate:** Several steps in this practice are adapted from a practice taught to me by therapist Marti Glenn, PhD, which she calls *vagal nurturing.* Here, I've added additional steps based on the latest neuroscience to add to this exercise's ability to specifically bring us out of the state of rumination.

Chapter 9: Neuroscience-Based Journaling Techniques

115 **"It would be nice to have":** Ben Stiller and Adam Scott, hosts, *The Severance Podcast with Ben Stiller and Adam Scott,* season 2, episode 6, "Attila," Audacy Podcasts, February 21, 2025.

116 **Researchers found that when we write:** F. R. van der Weel and A. L. H. van der Meer, "Handwriting but Not Typewriting Leads to Widespread Brain Connectivity: A High-Density EEG Study with Implications for the Classroom," *Frontiers in Psychology* 14 (2024): 1219945.

116 **Typing on digital devices:** P. Delgado et al., "Don't Throw Away Your Printed Books: A Meta-analysis on the Effects of Reading Media on Reading Comprehension," *Educational Research Review* 25 (November 2018): 23–28.

116 **He wondered if unprocessed stress:** James W. Pennebaker, *Opening Up: The Healing Power of Expressing Emotions* (Guilford Press, 1990), 23; J. Baranow et al. eds., *The Healing Art of Writing* (UC Medical Humanities Consortium, 2011), 3–4.

118 **They also required fewer:** J. W. Pennebaker et al., "Disclosure of Traumas and Immune Function: Health Implications for Psychotherapy," *Journal of Consulting and Clinical Psychology* 56, no. 2 (1988): 239–45.

118 **And in one follow-up study:** J. M. Smyth et al., "Effects of Writing About Stressful Experiences on Symptom Reduction in Patients with Asthma or Rheumatoid Arthritis: A Randomized Trial," *JAMA* 281, no. 14 (1999).

118 **Highly expressive individuals:** J. W. Pennebaker and S. K. Beall, "Confronting a Traumatic Event: Toward an Understanding of Inhibition and Disease," *Journal of Abnormal Psychology* 95, no. 3 (1986): 274–81.

119 **Duke researchers found that:** O. Glass et al., "Expressive Writing to Improve Resilience to Trauma: A Clinical Feasibility Trial," *Complementary Therapies in Clinical Practice* 34 (February 2019): 240–46.

119 **Other researchers found in a 2020 study:** S. F. Allen et al., "Online Writing About Positive Life Experiences Reduces Depression and Perceived Stress Reactivity in Socially Inhibited Individuals," *Psychiatry Research* 284 (February 2020): 112697.

121 **In a 2020 study, psychologists expanded:** H. Yang and H. Li, "Training Positive Rumination in Expressive Writing to Enhance Psychological

Adjustment and Working Memory Updating for Maladaptive Ruminators," *Frontiers in Psychology* 11 (May 2020): 789.

124 **Educational psychologist Kristin Neff:** K. D. Neff and C. Germer, "Self-Compassion and Psychological Wellbeing," chap. 27 in *Oxford Handbook of Compassion Science*, ed. J. Doty (Oxford University Press, 2017), 29.

124 **In one study of war veterans:** R. Hiraoka et al., "Self-Compassion as a Prospective Predictor of PTSD Symptom Severity Among Trauma-Exposed U.S. Iraq and Afghanistan War Veterans," *Journal of Traumatic Stress* 28, no. 2 (2015): 127–33; K. D. Neff et al., "Mindfulness, Self-Compassion, Posttraumatic Stress Disorder Symptoms, and Functional Disability in U.S. Iraq and Afghanistan War Veterans," *Journal of Traumatic Stress* 28, no. 5 (2015): 460–64.

125 **As Suleika Jaouad put it:** Elisabeth Egan, "Journaling Her Way Through Cancer for the Third Time," *New York Times*, April 19, 2025.

125 **If you love writing as a healing modality:** Mel Robbins, host, *The Mel Robbins Podcast*, "#1 Neurosurgeon: How to Manifest Anything You Want & Unlock the Unlimited Power of Your Mind," SiriusXM Podcasts, October 24, 2024.

126 **"I don't know how I would have managed":** Egan, "Journaling Her Way."

Chapter 10: Let the Positive Do Battle with the Negative—and Win!

128 **In a 2023 study, psychologists at Oregon:** H. R. Lawrence et al., "Reimagining Rumination? The Unique Role of Mental Imagery in Adolescents' Affective and Physiological Response to Rumination and Distraction," *Journal of Affective Disorders* 329 (May 2023): 460–69.

131 **First, studies show that each time:** K. Baumi et al., "Reinstating Memories' Temporal Context at Encoding Causes Sisyphus-Like Memory Rejuvenation," *Psychological and Cognitive Sciences* 122, no. 32 (2025): e2505120122.

135 **EMDR, or Eye Movement:** P. Manfied et al., "Use of Flash Technique in EMDR Therapy: Four Case Examples," *Journal of EMDR Practice and Research* 11, no. 4 (2017): 195–205.

143 **Over coffee, Paola demonstrates:** You can learn more about sociologist Martha Beck's work in her book *Finding Your Own North Star: Claiming the Life You Were Meant to Live* (Crown, 2002), 160. Also see Mel Robbins, host, *The Mel Robbins Podcast*, "How to Find Your Purpose & Design the Life You Want," SiriusXM Podcasts, January 23, 2025.

Chapter 11: The Power of Rest to Free You from Your Overthinking

146 **The clamor of our media-driven world:** C. S. Lewis, "Learning in War-Time," in *The Weight of Glory and Other Addresses* (HarperOne, 2001), 50.

147 **This serves as an excellent tool:** Christina Caron, "Are You a 'Floor Person'? Why Lying on the Ground Feels So Good," *New York Times*, March 8, 2024.

148 **In one study of fifty-four female:** A. Hassan and Z. Dshun, "Nature's Therapeutic Power: A Study on the Psychological Effects of Touching Ornamental Grass in Chinese Women," *Journal of Health, Population and Nutrition* 43, no. 1 (2024): 23.

150 **In one study of eighteen thousand people:** Claudia Hammond and Gemma Lewis, "The Rest Test: Preliminary Findings from a Large-Scale International Survey on Rest," chap. 8 in *The Restless Compendium: Interdisciplinary Investigations of Rest and Its Opposites*, ed. R. Callard, K. Staines, and J. Wilkes (Palgrave Macmillan, 2016).

151 **Both Albert Einstein and:** Nancy Andreasen, *The Creating Brain: The Neuroscience of Genius* (Dana Forlag, 2005), 120.

151 **She studied what happens to the brain:** Andreasen, *Creating Brain*, 73.

151 **Non-sleep deep rest:** O. Boukhris et al., "The Acute Effects of Non-sleep Deep Rest on Perceptual Responses, Physical, and Cognitive Performance in Physically Active Participants," *Applied Psychology: Health and Well Being* 16, no. 4 (2016): 1967–87; K. Delta et al., "Improved Sleep, Cognitive Processing and Enhanced Learning and Memory Task Accuracy with Yoga Nidra Practice in Novices," *PLOS One* 18, no. 12 (2023): e0294678.

152 **Boothroyd, whose online practices:** "Yoga Nidra for Deep Relaxation," YouTube video, 26:53, posted by Ally Boothroyd, March 3, 2025, https://www.youtube.com/watch?v=yj973M6ifB4.

153 **One aside here:** J. M. Newby et al., "Understanding the Experience of Rumination and Worry: A Descriptive Qualitative Survey Study," *British Journal of Clinical Psychology* 61, no. 4 (2022): 929–46.

153 **When you practice NSDR:** Laura Araujo, "How NSDR Combats Overstimulation and May Be the Key to Improving Your Cognitive Function," Maps Institute, May 26, 2021, https://themapsinstitute.com/how-nsdr-combats-overstimulation-and-may-be-the-key-to-improving-your-cognitive-function/.

153 **Feel-good, healthy hormones:** T. W. Kjaer et al., "Increased Dopamine Tone During Meditation-Induced Change of Consciousness," *Cognitive Brain Research* 13, no. 2 (2002): 255–59.

153 **And if you get this kind:** M. A. Immink, "Post-Training Meditation

Promotes Motor Memory Consolidation," *Frontiers in Psychology* 7 (October 2016): 1696.

153 **Researchers at the Laureate Institute:** Manoush Zomorodi et al., "Overwhelmed by Doom Scrolling? Time to Check in with Your Body," *TED Radio Hour*, NPR, October 31, 2023, https://www.npr.org/2023/10/31/1200611639/how-information-overload-impacts-our-mental-health.

154 **Floating in a sensory deprivation tank:** K. Jonsson and A. Kjellgren, "Promising Effects of Treatment with Flotation—REST (Restricted Environmental Stimulation Technique) as an Intervention for Generalized Anxiety Disorder (GAD): A Randomized Controlled Pilot Trial," *BMC Complementary and Alternative Medicine* 16 (March 2016): 108.

155 **This, in turn, helped veterans:** A. P. King et al., "Altered Default Mode Network (DMN) Resting State Functional Connectivity Following a Mindfulness-Based Exposure Therapy for Posttraumatic Stress Disorder (PTSD) in Combat Veterans of Afghanistan and Iraq," *Depression and Anxiety* 33, no. 4 (2016): 289–99.

155 **The Wheel of Awareness:** A. Villamil et al., "Cultivating Well-Being Through the Three Pillars of Mind Training: Understanding How Training the Mind Improves Physiological and Psychological Well-Being," *OBM Integrative and Complementary Medicine* 4, no. 1 (2019).

Chapter 12: When You Need More Help

161 **Multiple studies show that the degree:** T. Michael et al., "Rumination in Posttraumatic Stress Disorder," *Depression and Anxiety* 24, no. 5 (2007): 307–17; Y. Z. Szabo et al., "Rumination and Posttraumatic Stress Symptoms in Trauma-Exposed Adults: A Systematic Review and Meta-analysis," *Anxiety, Stress, and Coping* 30, no. 4 (2017): 396–414.

161 **Susan Nolen-Hoeksema at Yale:** "Most Women Think Too Much, Overthinkers Often Drink Too Much," *University of Michigan News*, February 4, 2003, https://news.umich.edu/most-women-think-too-much-overthinkers-often-drink-too-much/; D. P. Johnson and M. A. Whisman, "Gender Differences in Rumination: A Meta-analysis," *Personality and Individual Differences* 55, no. 4 (2013): 367–74.

161 **This gender difference emerges:** Johnson and Whisman, "Gender Differences."

161 **Due to differences in how:** Donna Jackson Nakazawa, *Girls on the Brink* (Harmony, 2022).

161 **Women also have to move through the world:** *Violence Against Women Prevalence Estimates, 2018* (World Health Organization, 2021).

162 **"I lost all sense of myself":** S. Arabi, "PTSD Symptoms: Romantic Relationships with Individuals Who Have Narcissistic and Psychopathic Traits" (master's thesis, Harvard University Division of Continuing Education, 2022).

162 **Researchers who examine the relationship:** R. A. Sansone and L. A. Sansone, "Rumination: Relationships with Physical Health," *Innovations in Clinical Neuroscience* 9, no. 2 (2012): 29–34; J. M. Newby et al., "Intrusive Thoughts and Images in Health Anxiety: Rates, Characteristics, and Responses," *Clinical Psychology and Psychotherapy* 31, no. 6 (2024): e70017.

162 **Happily, study after study:** G. Kokonyei et al., "Anticipation and Violated Expectation of Pain Are Influenced by Trait Rumination: An fMRI Study," *Cognitive, Affective, and Behavioral Neuroscience* 19, no. 1 (2019): 56–72.

165 **Over Zoom, Lanius shows me:** R. A. Lanius et al., "Reduced Cerebello-Thalamo-Cortical Functional Connectivity During Traumatic Memory Retrieval in PTSD," *Nature Mental Health*, in review.

165 **In a separate 2023 randomized:** R. A. Lanius et al., "A Randomized Controlled Trial of Deep Brain Reorienting: A Neuroscientifically Guided Treatment for Post-Traumatic Stress Disorder," *European Journal of Psychotraumatology* 14, no. 2 (2023): 2240691.

172 **A recent survey in the journal *Brain Stimulation:*** Charlotte Hu, "Are We Entering a Neurotechnology Renaissance in Healthcare?," Healthcare Brew, November 22, 2024, https://www.healthcare-brew.com/stories/2024/11/22/are-we-entering-neurotechnology-renaissance-healthcare.

173 **In a 2024 study, researchers showed that:** J. Pena et al., "Enhancement of Divergent Creative Thinking After Transcranial Near-Infrared Photobiomodulation over the Default Mode Network," *Creativity Research Journal* 36, no. 1 (2024): 1–14.

174 **A 2022 study by researchers:** T. Barba et al., "Effects of Psilocybin versus Escitalopram on Rumination and Thought Suppression in Depression," *British Journal of Psychiatry Open* 8, no. 5 (2022): e163.

175 **A 2023 study showed that using psychedelics:** J. J. Gattuso et al., "Default Mode Network Modulation by Psychedelics: A Systematic Review," *International Journal of Neuropsychopharmacology* 26, no. 3 (2023): 155–88.

175 **It creates changes in the default mode network:** R. A. Lanius, "The Sense of Self in the Aftermath of Trauma: Lessons from the Default Mode Network in Posttraumatic Stress Disorder," *European Journal of Psychotraumatology* 11, no. 1 (2020): 1807703.

175 **Ketamine has also been shown:** N. Zacharias et al., "Ketamine Effects on Default Mode Network Activity and Vigilance: A Randomized, Placebo-Controlled Crossover Simultaneous fMRI/EEG Study," *Human Brain Mapping* 41, no. 1 (2020): 107–19.

175 **All of these, she tells me:** Lanius, "The Sense of Self."

Chapter 13: The Upside of Rumination

179 **"You only have one mind and":** Ezra Klein, host, *The Ezra Klein Show*, podcast, "Marilynne Robinson on Biblical Beauty, Human Evil, and the Idea of Israel," *New York Times*, March 5, 2024.

191 **The French philosopher Simone Weil:** Simone Weil, *Waiting on God*, trans. Emma Craufurd (Harper & Row, 1951).

191 **Psychologist Mihaly Csikszentmihalyi:** Mihaly Csikszentmihalyi, *Creativity: Flow and the Psychology of Discovery and Invention* (Harper Perennial, 1997), 1.

191 **There is a good reason why:** *Merriam-Webster Dictionary*, "ruminate," https://www.merriam-webster.com/dictionary/ruminate.

191 **In 1822, Marie-Henri Beyle:** Stendhal, *On Love*, trans. Philip Sidney Woolf and Cecil N. Sidney Woolf (Brentano's, 1915). Originally published as *De l'amour* (Paris, 1822).

192 **"I believe in rumination":** Anaïs Nin, *Fire: From "A Journal of Love": The Unexpurgated Diary of Anaïs Nin, 1934–1937* (Brace, 1995).

192 **"many months in apparently":** Justin Morrow, "Watch: Daniel Day-Lewis on 'There Will Be Blood' and the Birth of an Infamous American Character," No Film School, July 19 2017, https://nofilmschool.com/2017/07/daniel-day-lewis-method-acting-there-will-be-blood-charlie-rose-interview#.

193 **This includes "daydreaming, planning for the future":** These quotes are taken from a short post written by Scott Barry Kaufman, which he shared on X on October 20, 2023. For more, see Scott Barry Kaufman, *Wired to Create: Unraveling the Mysteries of the Creative Mind* (Perigee, 2015). Also see S. B. Kaufman et al., "Default and Executive Network Coupling Supports Creative Idea Production," *Scientific Reports* 5 (June 2015): 10964.

193 **Big differences emerged:** S. B. Kaufman et al., "Differences in Brain Activity Patterns During Creative Idea Generation Between Eminent and Non-Eminent Thinkers," *NeuroImage* 220 (October 2020): 117011.

194 **Similarly, researchers at the University of North Carolina:** R. E. Beaty et al., "Creativity and the Default Network: A Functional Connectivity Analysis of the Creative Brain at Rest," *Neuropsychologia* 64 (2014): 92–98.

194 **She also talked about how being an actress:** Terry Gross, host, *Fresh Air*, podcast, "Emma Stone," NPR, January 31, 2024.

Chapter 14: What Does It Look Like When We Get Out of Our Own Way?

197 **Kaufman, like Singer, argues:** S. B. Kaufman et al., "Ode to Positive Constructive Daydreaming," *Frontiers in Psychology* 23, no. 4 (2013): 626.

198 **Letting your daydreams flow:** Kristin Weir, "The Science Behind Creativity," *Monitor on Psychology* 53, no. 3 (2022): 40.

198 **Gopnik likens this open, creative mental state:** Ezra Klein, host, *The Ezra Klein Show*, podcast, "Ezra Klein Interviews Alison Gopnik," *New York Times*, April 16, 2021. This is also based on my 2022 email exchanges with Gopnik. For more on this, see Gopnik's book *The Philosophical Baby* (Farrar, Straus and Giroux, 2009).

199 **"Creativity is a wild mind and a disciplined eye":** This quote is widely attributed to Dorothy Parker, including on Goodreads.com.

199 **Brian Eno, the inventor of:** Sean Illing interviewed philosopher Simon Critchley, where Critchley talked about a concept that Brian Eno, the inventor of generative music, calls "idiot glee." Sean Illing, host, *The Gray Area*, podcast, "The Case for Not Overthinking," Vox Media, December 9, 2024.

200 **Your brain starts to create:** J. Kounios et al., "Creative Flow as Optimized Processing: Evidence from Brain Oscillations During Jazz Improvisations by Expert and Non-Expert Musicians," *Neuropsychologia* 196 (2024): 108824.

200 **In one study using neuroimaging:** "Your Brain in the Zone: A New Neuroimaging Study Reveals How the Brain Achieves a Creative Flow State," *Science Daily*, March 4, 2024; J. Kounios et al., "Creative Flow as Optimized Processing."

201 **"If you start a song":** Rick Rubin, *The Creative Act: A Way of Being* (Penguin, 2023), 130.

203 **One of NASA's concerns:** Nathaniel Rich, "Can Humans Endure the Psychological Torment of Mars?," *New York Times*, February 25, 2024.

203 **Eventually, they lost their ability to focus:** Rich, "Can Humans Endure?"

203 **That "curiosity that draws you":** Weir, "The Science Behind Creativity."

203 **And yes—you know this science by now:** Scott Barry Kaufman and Carolyn Gregoire, "Ten Habits of Highly Creative People," *Greater Good Magazine*, January 20, 2016; S. B. Kaufman et al., "Personality and Complex Brain Networks: The Role of Openness to Experience

in Default Network Efficiency," *Human Brain Mapping* 37, no. 2 (2016): 773–79.

203 **Creativity is the ability to:** H. Gardner, "Commentary: Getting at the Heart of the Creative Experience," *LEARNing Landscapes* 6, no. 1 (2012): 45–54; "Howard Gardner on Creativity—Are Schools Encouraging Creativity? The Challenge of Creativity," *Leading and Learning,* October 31, 2023, https://leading-learning.blogspot.com/2013/10/howard-gardner-on-creativity-are.html; Sergey Markov, "Howard Gardner: Author of the Theory of Multiple Intelligences," *Genvive,* July 5, 2024, https://geniusrevive.com/en/howard-gardner-author-of-the-theory-of-multiple-intelligences-and-prominent-creativity-researcher/.

204 **It seems to me that:** Hannah Levintova, "Maria Popova's Beautiful Mind," *Mother Jones,* January/February 2012.

205 **Mihaly Csikszentmihalyi argues that:** Mihaly Csikszentmihalyi, *Creativity: Flow and the Psychology of Discovery and Invention* (HarperCollins, 1996), 73.

205 **L'Engle was inspired by:** Leonard S. Marcus, "Leonard S. Marcus on Madeleine L'Engle, the 'Fearless Experimenter' of Children's Literature," Library of America, October 19, 2018, https://www.loa.org/news-and-views/1445-leonard-s-marcus-on-madeleine-l8217engle-the-fearless-experimenter-of-childrens-literature/.

209 **If you want to play the piano:** Rachel Martin, "Rick Rubin on Taking Communion with Johnny Cash and Not Rushing Creativity," *All Things Considered,* NPR, December 10, 2023.

210 **(This brings to mind):** Rubin, *The Creative Act,* 78.

213 **"There is a multi-front war":** Sam Harris, host, *Making Sense with Sam Harris,* podcast, "Thoughts Without a Thinker," January 21, 2025.

214 **Ninety-one percent of participants:** Allison Aubrey, "A Break from Your Smartphone Can Reboot Your Mood. Here's How Long You Need," *Living Better,* NPR, February 24, 2025, https://www.npr.org/2025/02/24/nx-s1-5304417/smartphone-break-digital-detox-screen-addiction.

214 **Perhaps you remember the famous marshmallow:** W. Mischel and E. B. Ebbesen, "Attention in Delay of Gratification," *Journal of Personality and Social Psychology* 16, no. 2 (1970): 329–37.

214 **By finding constructive ways:** Alfie Kohn, "S'More Misrepresentation of Research," *Education Week,* September 10, 2014; Janine Zacharia, "The Bing 'Marshmallow Studies': 50 Years of Continuing Research," Stanford Bing Nursery School Distinguished Lecture Series, September 24, 2015, https://bingschool.stanford.edu/news/bing-marshmallow-studies-50-years-continuing-research.

215 **But here's what surprised me:** L. M. Hilt and S. D. Pollak, "Getting Out

of Rumination: Comparison of Three Brief Interventions in a Sample Youth," *Journal of Abnormal Child Psychology* 40, no. 7 (2012): 1157–65.

217 **For him, he says:** Weir, "The Science Behind Creativity."

217 **We become open to:** Rachel Kushner, *Creation Lake* (Scribner, 2024), 45–46.

217 **One strategy I use:** Jeremy Utley, "Hijack Your Subconscious Mind," Methods of the Masters, May 23, 2025, https://www.jeremyutley.design/blog/hijack-your-subconscious-mind.

219 **As he stood knee-deep in a flooded field:** David Whyte, *The Bell and the Blackbird* (Many Rivers Press, 2018).

219 **Combining walking with being in nature:** M. Oppezzo and D. L. Schwartz, "Give Your Ideas Some Legs: The Positive Effect of Walking on Creative Thinking," *Journal of Experimental Psychology: Learning, Memory, and Cognition* 40, no. 4 (2014): 1142–52.

219 **To use Nietzsche's words:** Friedrich Nietzsche, *Twilight of the Idols*, trans. R. J. Hollingdale (Penguin, 1990), 34.

220 **Awe removes us from our self-preoccupation:** Hope Reese, "How a Bit of Awe Can Improve Your Health," *New York Times*, January 3, 2023.

220 **Another study showed that college students:** L. Luo et al., "Awe Experience Triggered by Fighting Against COVID-19 Promotes Prosociality Through Increased Feeling of Connectedness and Empathy," *Journal of Positive Psychology* 18, no. 6 (2023): 866–82.

221 **Whenever my mind returns to:** Kathleen Rooney, "Kathleen Rooney on Rene Magritte's 'Selected Writings,'" Poetry Society of America, https://poetrysociety.org/poems-essays/in-their-own-words/kathleen-rooney-on-ren%C3%A9-magrittes-selected-writings.

Appendix: Are You Ruminating Too Much?

227 **In consultation with experts, including Ruth Lanius:** This questionnaire is not intended to be used as a diagnostic tool. It draws from my interviews with Ruth Lanius, MD, PhD, on how the default mode network is shaped by our challenging life experiences and can show up as negative, ruminative thought patterns in daily life. I've also drawn from assessments used by researchers in the field. For a more detailed, clinical assessment (which should be used in consultation with a behavioral health professional), see Rumination-Reflection Questionnaire (RRQ): P. D. Trapnell and J. D. Campbell, "Private Self-Consciousness and the Five-Factor Model of Personality: Distinguishing Rumination from Reflection," *Journal of Personality and Social Psychology* 76, no. 2 (1999): 284–304; and T. Ehring et al., "The Per-

severative Thinking Questionnaire (PTQ): Validation of a Content-Independent Measure of Repetitive Thinking," *Journal of Behavior Therapy and Experimental Psychiatry* 42, no. 2 (2011): 225–32. For quick pop psychology quizzes, you can find many online on platforms like Psychologia.

INDEX

A

B

K

L

M

O

P

S

U

V

W

Y

Z

ABOUT THE AUTHOR

Donna Jackson Nakazawa is the author of five books that examine the intersection of neurobiology, emotion, and mental health. Her book *Girls on the Brink: Helping Our Daughters Thrive in an Era of Increased Anxiety, Depression, and Social Media* was named one of the best health books of 2022 by *The Washington Post* and *Mashable.* Donna's other books include *The Angel and the Assassin: The Tiny Brain Cell That Changed the Course of Medicine,* named one of the best books of 2020 by *Wired* magazine, and *Childhood Disrupted,* a finalist for the Books for a Better Life Award. She's also the author of *The Adverse Childhood Experiences Guided Journal.* Her books have been translated into fifteen languages, attracting a worldwide audience.

Her writing has appeared in *Wired, The Boston Globe, Psychology Today, Psychotherapy Networker, Stat, The Washington Post,* and *Health Affairs.* She has appeared on the *Today* show and NPR and is a regular speaker at conferences and universities, including the Child Mind Institute, the Harvard Division of Science Library Series, UCLA Health, UCLA Open Mind, Rutgers University, Johns Hopkins, Children's Hospital Association, the Andrew Weil Center for Integrative Medicine at the University of Arizona, and hundreds of other institutions. Jackson Nakazawa is also the creator of the narrative writing-to-heal program Breaking Free from Trauma, which helps participants to create a new, powerful inner-healing narrative that calms the body, brain, and nervous system.

donnajacksonnakazawa.com